THE GEEZER'S GUIDE TO BETTER HEALTH AND LONGEVITY

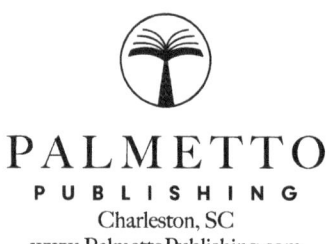

PALMETTO
PUBLISHING
Charleston, SC
www.PalmettoPublishing.com

Paperback ISBN: 9798822968639

THE GEEZER'S GUIDE TO BETTER HEALTH AND LONGEVITY

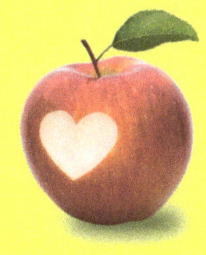

ALAN LARIVEE

Visit us on the web! geezersguide.org

Photos by Alan Larivee, Mike Herron, Dave Hamberg

Disclaimer: My intention in writing this small yet hopefully impactful book is to inform on many healthy diet concepts learned and actions taken over many decades, with hopes you will consider trying some of them and that by doing so you will become healthier and feel better. That written, just because this protocol works for me doesn't mean it will work for you. That is a true statement. People are physically different, so please consult with your doctor before you consume any foods or attempt any processes I present. And so I must unfortunately declare I may not be held accountable, though I hope you will at least appreciate the fact this disclaimer is printed in a readable font.

Also, anything you decide to attempt, please do so in small portions at first.

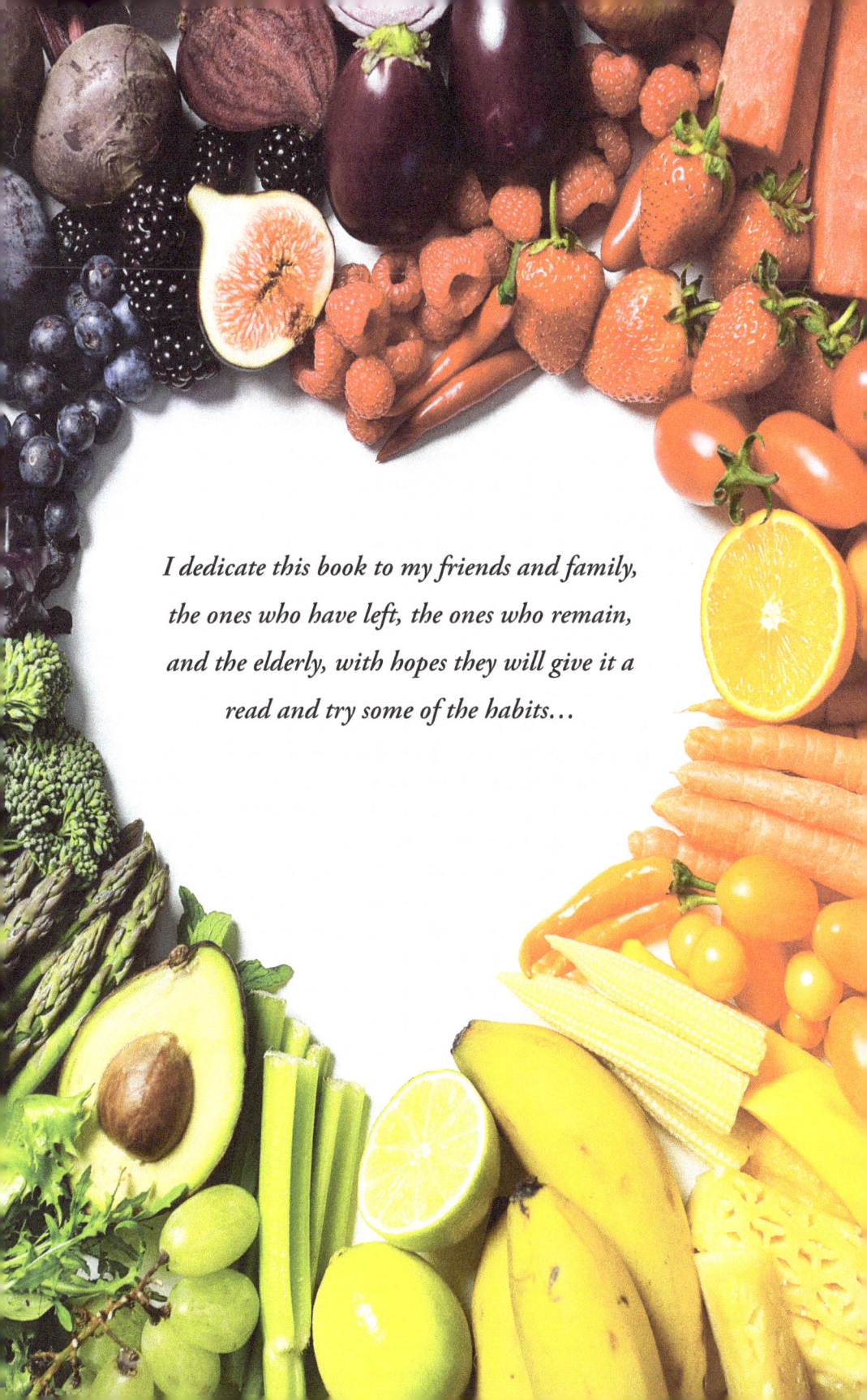

I dedicate this book to my friends and family,
the ones who have left, the ones who remain,
and the elderly, with hopes they will give it a
read and try some of the habits…

CONTENTS

THE GEEZER'S GUIDE: INTRODUCTION

I am a fixer by nature. If there is trash on the ground, I'll pick it up. If the shopping carts outside the grocery store are not in order, I'll set them straight. If there's something on the wall not level, I will level it. I can't help it—it's my nature. I am also a builder by occupation, but usually not new things. I prefer working on old things. I want to make them better.

Perhaps that's why, over many decades, I've studied and participated in many modern diet concepts. As new approaches to

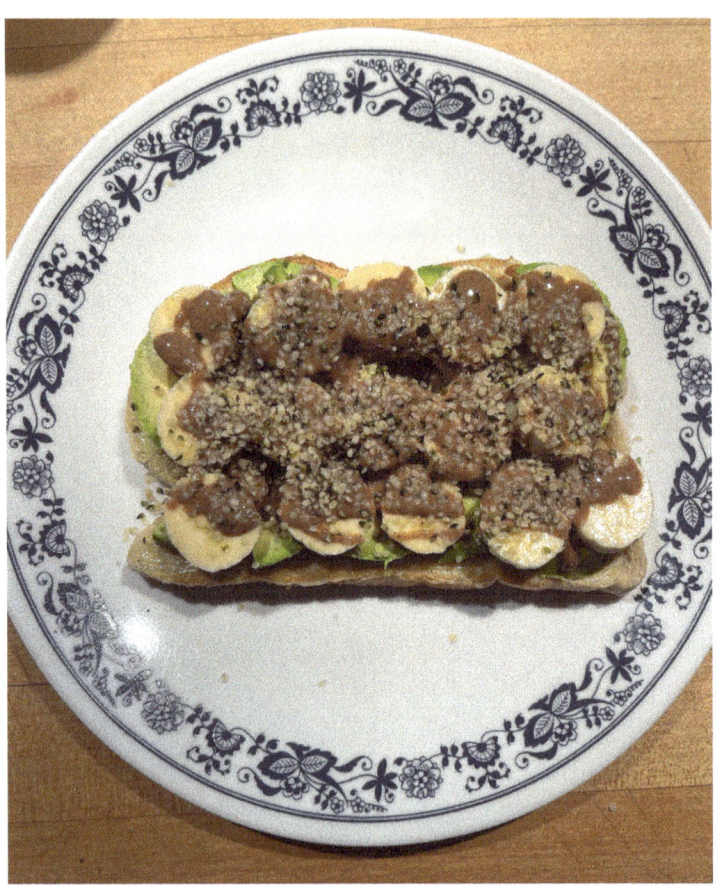

Avocado, banana, shelled hemp and almond butter on sourdough. Complete nutrition!

health and longevity evolve, so too does my fascination. And though I am now older, I still want to be better than the current standard of my age. I've gained information you may find helpful.

As I write these words, I am sixty-seven years old. I'm five foot, eleven inches tall and weigh 175 pounds. I see a doctor every year and am tested, yet I'm never prescribed medication. I'm occasionally told I'm still handsome—not true—but I do have lots of energy and my cognitive skills are still relatively sharp. I've never been diagnosed with a serious illness, never spent the night in a hospital bed.

In June of 2024, I had a standard physical with complete blood work: hemoglobin, PSA, TSH, vitamin, lipids, and so on. My doctor was satisfied with all my test results. She also described my kidney, liver, thyroid function and prostate as normal, no hepatitis, no diabetes and my blood pressure at the time of my visit was also within the normal standard. I figure I must be doing something right, though I do not profess *perfect* health. I am, of course, aging and there are genetic as well as sports-related issues, which I will relate later in the book, that I must address. Also, please consider I'm receiving positive results despite working over forty-five years in an occupation with notoriously toxic conditions (construction).

If you're reading this book, I figure you are at least in your fifties, probably in your sixties or seventies, perhaps eighties. (Anyone in their nineties in "good" condition needn't read further!) What I intend to do is convince you that most of the food you've been eating your entire life will no longer sustain you, that your aging physiology needs better nutrition. If you want to rid yourself of "diseases of the fork," you must add foods that will make you healthier and feel better, plus leave behind foods and habits your body can no longer tolerate. I have lost a lot of friends and family who, in their later years, became ill and would not alter their eating habits. They didn't believe eating better makes you healthier or were so entrenched with their dietary habits they couldn't stop. But it does make you healthier, so please let me to introduce the concepts and habits I have used for many years, which give me the positive results I have received. We must nurture our bodies—they're the only ones we've got!

As it is my intention to make this book as succinct as possible, I created three main sections: food additions, foods to omit, and some healthy habits to attempt that I've done for years. But first allow me to define *nutrition* in succinct form.

NUTRITION

Nutrition is the bodily process of obtaining the materials needed for a functional human stasis via the three major macronutrients:

1. **Carbohydrates**— "molecules of varying size and complexity that provide fuel for energy" (45) and brain function—basically carbon, hydrogen and oxygen that convert into the different saccharides.

2. **Protein**—specific configurations of twenty amino acids with nine essential (meaning the human body can't make them). There are over fifty thousand different types of proteins with different functions.

3. **Fats, or lipids**—like carbs, they are basically carbon, hydrogen, and oxygen (the difference being molecular configuration). Fats are a backup fuel source; there are unsaturated (healthiest type), saturated (mostly animal fats except coconuts), and trans fats (man-made, evil!). As needed, humans can convert protein into carbs or fat but cannot turn fat or carbs into protein.

Also needed are essential *micronutrients*, the necessary chemical elements or vitamins, substances that must be obtained through our diet, mainly carbon, hydrogen, oxygen, nitrogen, and sulfur (though there are many others); *blood builders*, such as iron, copper, cobalt, and so on; the *electrolytes*, such as potassium, magnesium, phosphates, and so on; the tens of thousands of different *enzymes*, our physiological worker agents that make everything happen; and *clean water* (45).

Though this simplest of definitions doesn't do justice to the complexity of human physiology and nutrition, thanks to Barry Sears, who wrote *Enter the Zone*, before I eat any meal, I ask myself if the meal I'm about to consume is giving me proper nutrition: the fats, protein and carbohydrates, as well as essential minerals (1).

DANGED CHEMISTRY

I have found it amazing how in all the dozens of health and longevity books I have read through the years, few ever give simple explanations on their scientific terminology. But if you want to write about nutrition, you must enter into a science complex and baffling to most. I am nothing close to a chemist, but I have spent many years reading books that have helped me figure out a lot of chemistry terminology and will parenthesize definitions when necessary. Also please know that I won't be creating any *Geezers* T-shirts or ball caps and won't become some evolved swami or expert on everything under the sun because I wrote a book. I'm interested in making old folks healthier, that's all.

So let's go!

FOODS TO ADD

HEALTHY FATS

Do *not* fear fats! At least do not fear the healthy ones. My favorites are olive, avocado and MCT oil. Like avocados, olives are composed of oleic acid. These monounsaturated fats will lower high cholesterol levels and have healing and anti-inflammatory properties (3). MCT oil (medium chain triglycerides) are, according to Dr. Gundry's *The Plant Paradox*, a necessary component to a healthy fat health protocol. MCTs are highly biologically accessible fats that easily convert to energy. MCTs, olive oil and avocado oil are the best fats for human consumption!

Walmart sells the Carrington Farms brand MCT oil powder that can be purchased in large five-ounce bags or twelve go-packs. I will occasionally sprinkle a heaping teaspoon on gluten-free cereal instead of sugar. The go-packs I use as an occasional

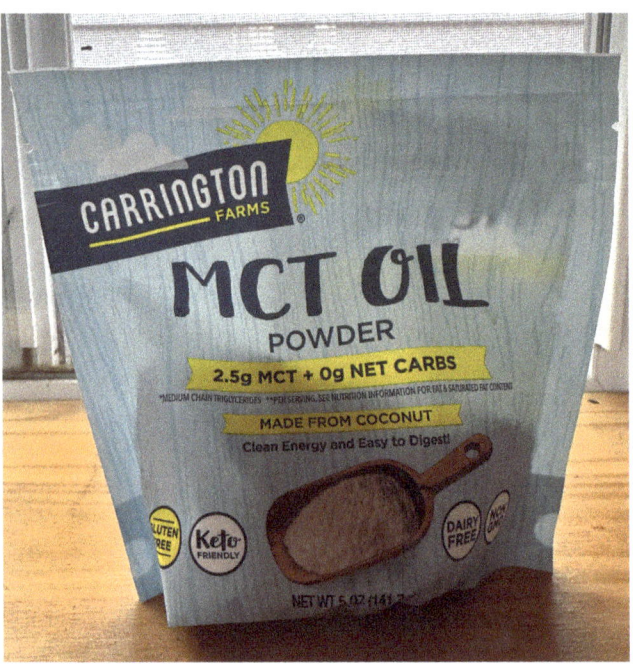

pick-me-up. I just pour it in my mouth and wash it down with water; it actually tastes good. Fats are foods that last and keep our systems satisfied. Carbs burn fast, while fats burn slower and keep working longer.

Guacamole is my favorite food and a very healthy food choice. It's made with avocados, root vegetables, onion and garlic; even blood-purifying cilantro. And being a true avocado whisperer, I can tell you how to purchase and create the perfect avocado. Buy your avocados green, as the ripe ones in the store are often bruised. Take them home and put them in a large brown paper bag, shutting the top with a clothespin or two. Wait two or three days, then take one out of the bag and feel it. If the avocado's skin gives slightly, it may be ready. Gently tap the avocado on your kitchen counter. A deep sound on the bump suggests a ripe avocado. Cut the avocado around the very large seed. If you're able to pull it apart, it's probably ripe. If not, wrap it in BPA-free wrapping and put it back in the bag. I must admit it's rare, but sometimes avocados don't ripen; they stay hard and green. They're expensive and you feel cheated. My apologies beforehand.

"Coconuts can save your life," declares David Wolfe in his book *Eating for Beauty*. I have religiously consumed coconut products for at least twenty years in the form of cream, water, and oil. Unlike the long-chain saturated fatty acids derived from animal fats, coconut oil's medium-chain saturated fatty acids provide health benefits, contain antioxidants, support healthy hormone production, help displace toxic hydrogenated fats, support heart health and help control blood sugar levels (4). I put coconut oil on my skin to replenish it and I eat the cream to remain nutritiously oiled. Coconut water is the liquid component for my morning drink.

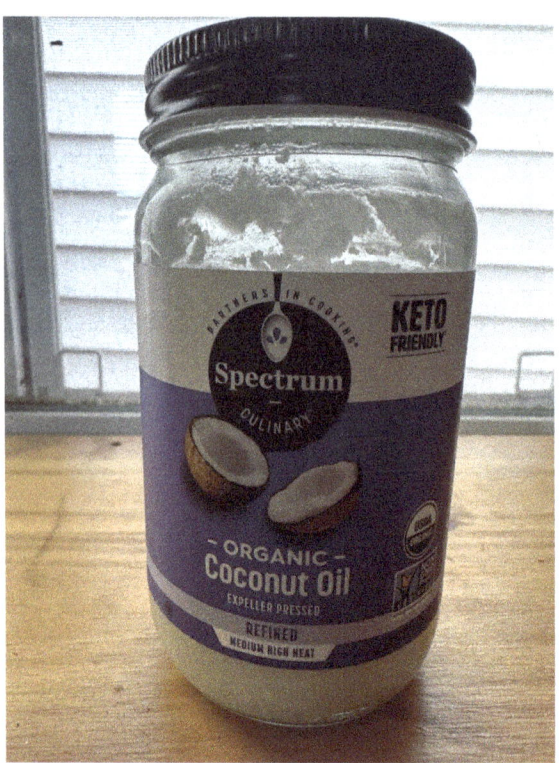

Note: When eating fats, it is beneficial to take the enzyme lipase to assist fat digestion. I will cover enzyme nutrition further in the book.

This is a recipe I use often. It comes from the book *Eat Fat to Lose Fat* by Mary Enig and Sally Fallon.

Mary's Oil Blend

1/3 cup coconut oil

1/3 cup olive oil

1/3 cup sesame oil

Warm the coconut oil slightly, just enough to liquify it, as coconut oil is solid until seventy-six degrees or above. Mix all the oils together. If the blend solidifies, put in a tad more olive oil.

This is a great all-use oil for cooking, drizzling on salads, and whenever you need oil (35).

Also please consider the *light* use of clarified butter (or ghee) in place of regular butter or margarine. Ghee is lactose-free, nutritionally dense, loaded with omega-3 fatty acids, is more digestible and is user-friendly as it spreads easier than butter (33), though at home I usually pour avocado oil on my toast, as I consider it the healthiest choice. Monounsaturated fats are best (64).

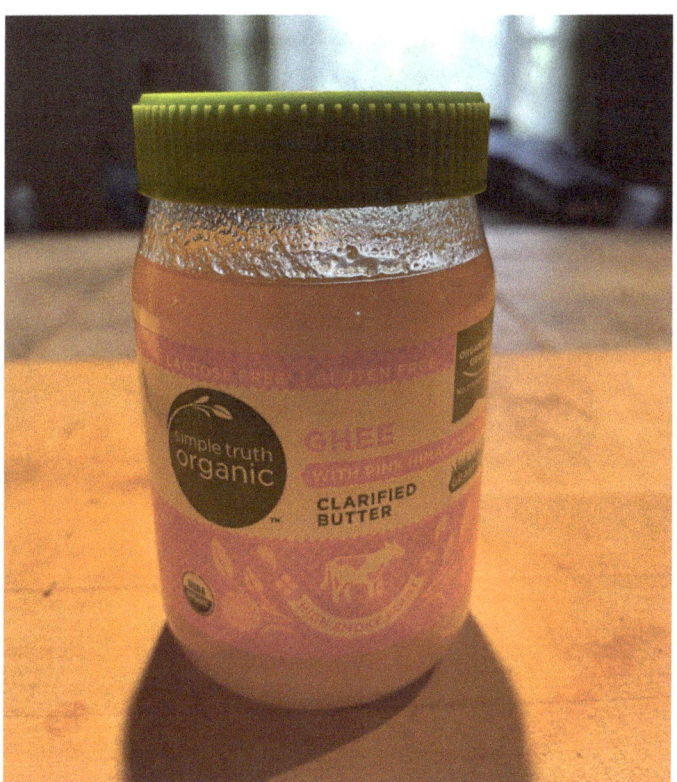

CACAO

The cacao to which I refer is raw chocolate in its most basic form, known in antiquity as *the food of the gods*. And who can argue? There's something about chocolate that's…indescribably wonderful! And to think, it's one of the world's most nutritiously packed foods when consumed correctly. When I began consuming raw cacao, my health improved.

Spanish explorer Hernan Cortez learned of cacao from the Aztecs, who called cacao *heart blood*, which makes sense, as cacao is a heart-healthy food (2). Its antioxidant value *far exceeds* any other food and is stocked with many beneficial and crucial elements, including copper, zinc, magnesium, iron and the amino acid tryptophan, necessary for the production of the

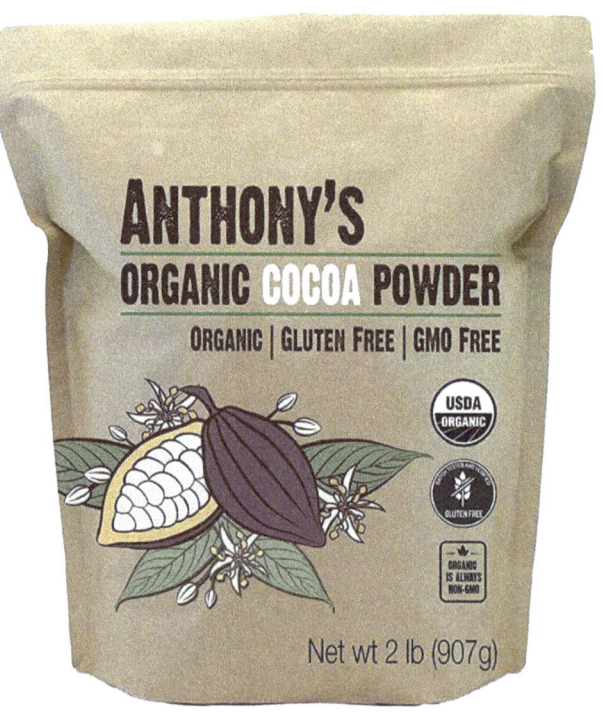

mood-modulating neurotransmitter serotonin, which helps humans feel relaxed. It also contains theobromine (an alkaloid) that opens the bloodstream and reduces blood pressure, making the heart's job simpler (38).

I consume raw cacao in my morning drink. I use cacao nibs, as I like to crunch them, though most folks use the powder form for smoothies. I also consume dark chocolate bars at lunch. I go for the high percentage (78 percent or better) with a small serving size. Cacao is a terrific mood enhancer that helps with depression (46). It lifts my spirits and occasionally causes me to do a sort of silly dance, behaving as if I had rhythm.

I have all sorts of healthy foods in my fridge. None is healthier than cacao.

BONE BROTH PROTEIN

When your bones weaken, you lose strength, so most every year I take a Lifeline Screening test. This company travels from town to town; they administer certain tests, such as aortic sonograms, blood tests and so on. I started doing this after my health insurance company dropped me for no apparent reason other than, I must assume, I was getting too old for coverage. So I took these screenings which I could afford. For the first couple of years my tests came back fine for me with the exception of *bone density*. I was losing bone mass. And since osteoporosis was not mentioned in my DNA results, I assumed the cause may be related to my occupation, as well as general environmental toxicity from air and water. It was several years later, when I was able to receive health care again, that I was able to show my doctor my screening

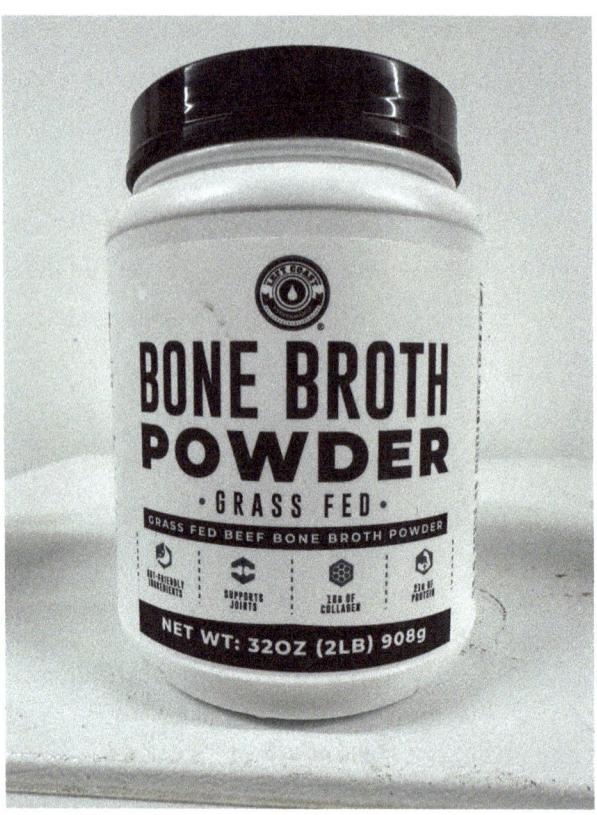

results. My doctor suggested I buy meat bones from the butcher's shop, steam them in a pot and drink the broth. Since I practically live in health food stores and was aware of bone broth protein, I asked my doctor if I could try that instead, which I did. Since taking bone broth protein regularly, my *bone density* results have all been within standard range.

ALOE

This is one of David Wolfe's top ten *superfoods* and one of the most extraordinary plants on the planet, with vast healing properties. You name it, aloe vera does it. Stocked with vital minerals, it soothes the digestive tract, reduces inflammation (3) and has become an amazing addition to my health routine. At this writing, I have eleven aloe plants growing in my sunroom. One plant I've owned for several years, after using all of its leaves except a few small leaves still growing at the top of the plant, grew back after I chopped off the old trunk and stuck the leaves into potting soil!

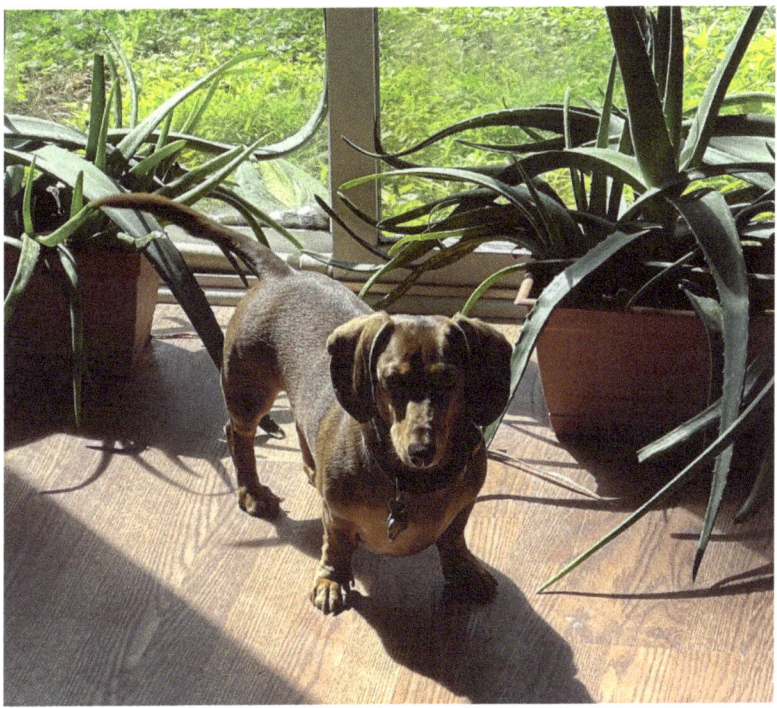

Mickey guarding the aloe plants.

You don't need to grow your own plants, however. All of my local food markets sell the leaves—probably true in your area as well. The way you consume aloe, depending on the thickness of the leaf, as the leaves are thick at the base and thin at the tips, is to cut three-fourths to one and a half inches from the leaf. From there, you either fillet the inner gel with a knife or (what I do) cut the edges off, slice the piece in half and rake the gel into your

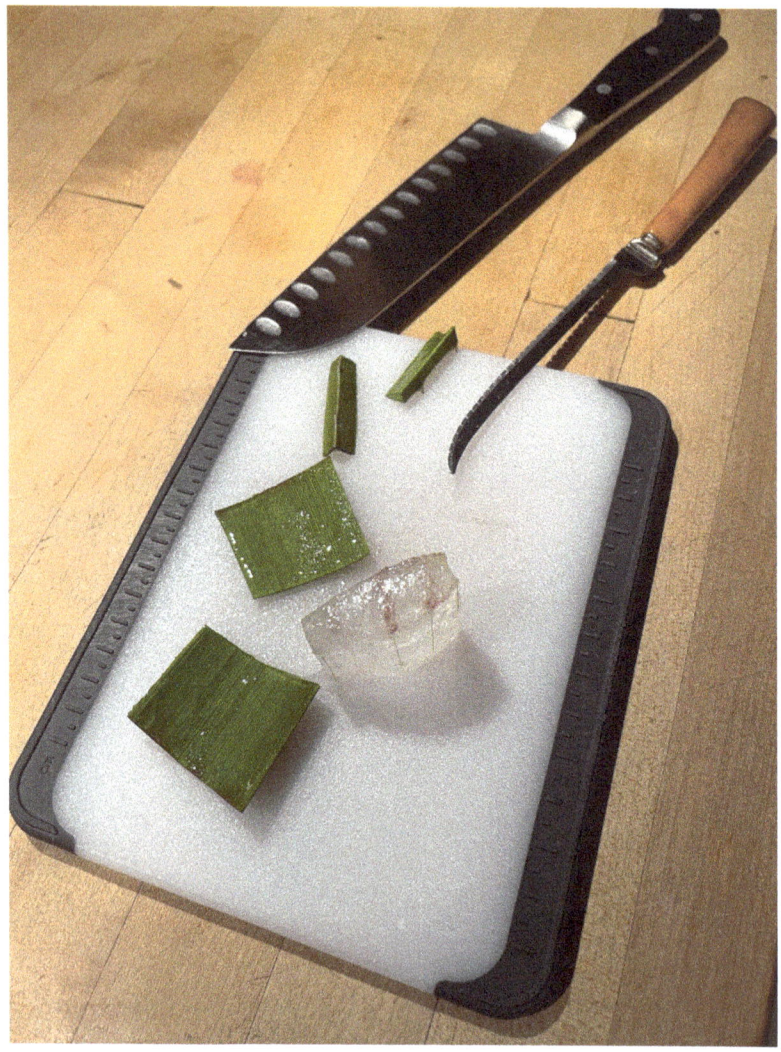

mouth with your teeth. Aloe has a very bitter taste. Frankly, it tastes awful. But when has medicine ever tasted good? Folks who consume aloe usually put it in smoothies, though I just slurp it down with warm water. Aloe also stimulates the bowels—not a bad thing first thing in the morning. It also helps regulate blood sugar and improves digestion (59). And try taking the inside of the aloe skin and rubbing the gel side on your face, arms, all over. Our skin is our largest organ and needs nourishment too!

In 2015, I received an awful sports injury and was hauled away in an ambulance. Luckily, X-rays showed nothing broken, but I had a black bruise running all along my lower back and down the back of both legs to my calves. I lay in bed for a week, performed hot-to-cold hydrotherapy in the shower and applied aloe all over my bruised area several times a day. After a week or so, I was back on my feet after using this method.

Like so many fellas, as I got into my fifties, I found my-self having to pee two, three times every night. Since consuming aloe, I don't have that problem.

COLOSTRUM

A while back, while watching a nutrition podcast, I was intro-duced to a man named Daniel Vitalis, a naturalist living up in Maine whose back-to-nature message spoke truth to me. I went to his website, SurThrival.com, where I was introduced to bovine colostrum. Female mammals, after giving birth but before feed-ing their newborns milk, release colostrum to feed their babies as an immunity activation. Colostrum greatly strengthens the im-mune system, improves gut health, helps repair tissue, increases stamina and brain function (18). I have been taking colostrum for many years, practically every day. I am very seldom sick.

Colostrum is a superfood of the umpteenth degree and the main ingredient of my morning drink. I highly recommend its use.

MACA ROOT AND CAMU CAMU BERRY

These are four other amazing ingredients I also consume in my morning drink. *Maca* is grown in the high Andes mountains and is known for its great health qualities, including the following:

1. Energy and endurance

2. Mood enhancing

3. Improves memory

4. Fights free radicals

5. Lowers blood pressure (62).

(Folks with thyroid issues should omit.)

Here's what's great about camu camu berry:

- Highest known source of raw vitamin C
- High in antioxidants
- Anti-inflammatory
- Anti-microbial
- Improves blood sugar (64).

BEE POLLEN AND CHLORELLA

Super green chlorella:

High in B-12 (Making meat/dairy consumption unnecessary.)
High in omega 3's.
Detoxifier - Binds to heavy metals; weakens metal toxicity
in organs.
Enhances immune system (65).

And Bee pollen:

Super nutrient rich!
Supports immune system.
Supports natural detoxification.
Supports appropriate blood sugar levels and metabolic
function (66).

Because of their amazing degree of health composition, these
four ingredients go in the morning drink.

HOLISTIC TINCTURES

For many years, I have regularly purchased health products from the American Botanical Pharmacy website. The products, created by Dr. Richard Schulze, must run under the category *industrial strength*. You consume it, it works. The tinctures I use regularly—Brain, Cayenne, and SuperFood PLUS powder—work as succinctly as their product names. They work like the no-crap, *give-it-to-me-straight* demeanor of their creator. (Look him up; his videos are great.)

In early 2022, a friend and I started feeling a tad off with a general weakness and soreness. Thinking it may be COVID, I hit Dr. Schulze' Cayenne Tincture and Superfood Plus hard. My friend lay in bed for several days while I kept working, though I stayed away from others. On another occasion, a friend was feeling rough, so I brought over a bottle of ABP's SuperTonic, the *all-purpose miracle tonic*, to save him and save him it did. For whatever reason you feel yourself lacking, give the appropriate tincture or product a try. This stuff works.

CANNABINOL TINCTURES

A few years back, I noticed a new store at the strip center next the Butts Station railroad tracks named *Hemp Haven*. Since I was familiar with shelled hemp and the store was close to home, I decided to check it out. The proprietor patiently described her many fascinating products: tinctures, oils, gummies, products for people and pets. I veered away from the THC products (never liked being stoned) but was very interested in the anti-inflammatory properties of the tinctures. After some discussion, it was decided a CBD/CBG tincture was right for me. "Study suggests CBD-rich treatment has a beneficial impact on pain, anxiety and depression symptoms as well as overall well being…" (56).

Cannabinol tinctures are part of my health protocol. The science of cannabinols is relatively new. I believe there will be many more longevity-inducing products derived from the hemp plant.

FERMENTED VEGETABLES

This habit I adopted from Donna Gates's *The Body Ecology Diet*. Though the practice of fermenting vegetables in the far east and northern Europe is quite old, it's become popular in present-day America. (For the unfamiliar, this stuff is coleslaw that's been fermented; it's the original coleslaw!) Consuming fermented veggies creates healthy gut flora for the intestinal tract. They are also packed with digestive enzymes (30). For years, I bought the correct bacterial strain from the *Body Ecology* website and would take the better part of the morning running veggies through my Grandmaw's late '70s food processor, making enough vegetables to last three months. Then one day, as I walked through the grocery store, I was surprised to find bags and jars of fermented vegetables. I bought a bag, took it home and was a tad upset to find it tasted better than mine, though since then I've cranked up on the onions and garlic to improve. The point here is you don't have to make your own. Fermented vegetables go in *all* my homemade salads.

Here are some of the ingredients I use to create fermented veggies. Cabbage, carrots, garlic and onions are my basic mainstays. The other ingredients I use occasionally include kale, ginger, celery, apples, lemons and dulse (a type of seaweed—mineral rich!).

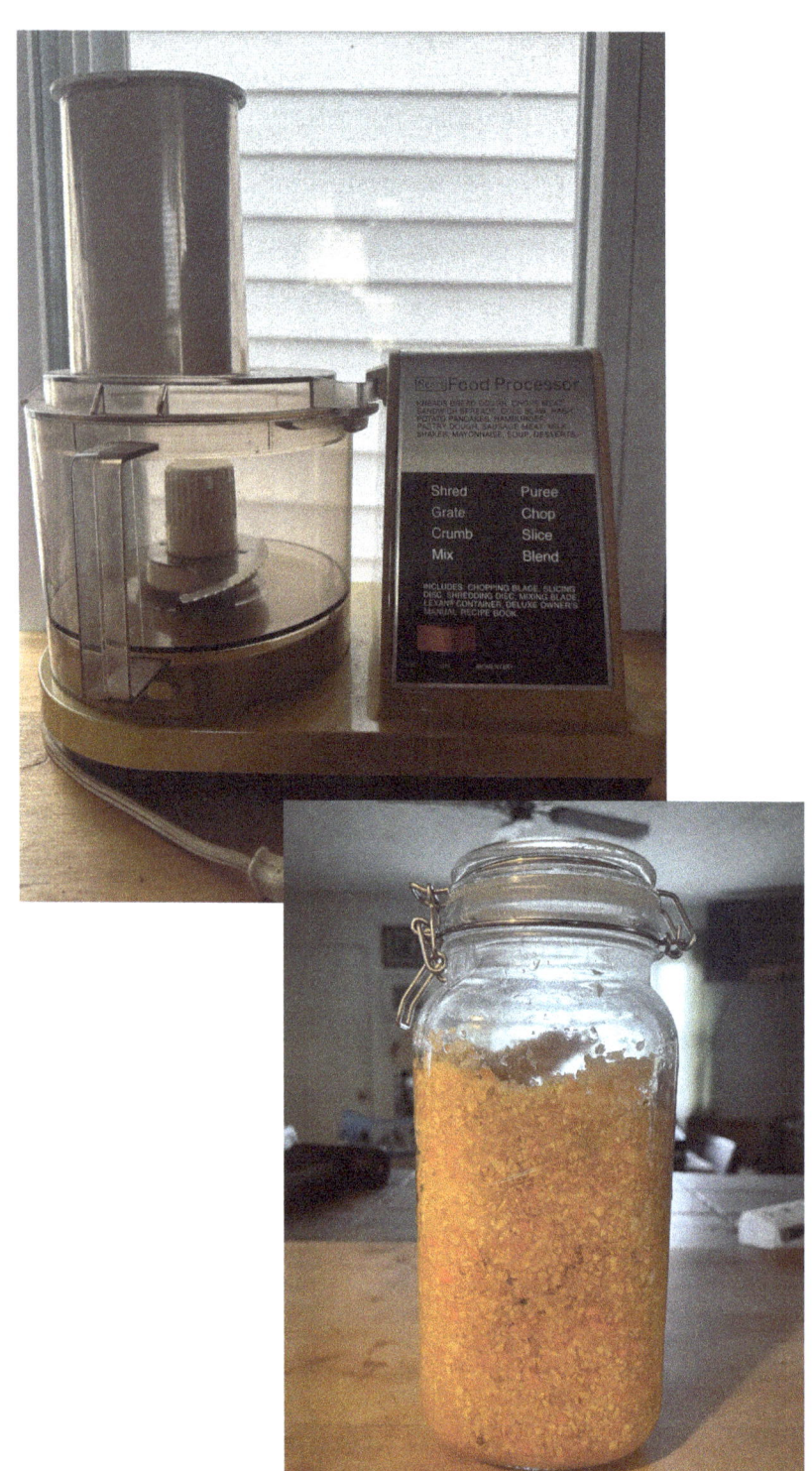

RAW SALADS

While reading Dr. Jensen's *Guide to Body Chemistry and Nutrition*, I noticed how so many essential trace minerals come from plain raw greens, an unacknowledged superfood. My salad consists mainly of organic greens, whenever available. A personal favorite is Living Lettuce, easy-to-chew butter lettuce set in containers that allow roots, still intact. Take it easy on the roughage, specifically the so-called *super greens*, as they may be difficult for geezers to chew and digest, though the typical spring mix doesn't seem too rough. And I like spinach, as it's a soft chew and it's super dark-green color suggests optimal nutrition, though I switch between different types of greens, as spinach contains oxalic acid, which may produce kidney stones (67). Avoid or tweak (remove the seeds from) from veggies like tomatoes and cucumbers, as their seeds contain lectins, which, as reported in *The Plant Paradox*, permeate the gut lining. Go with root veggies like onions and radishes. Celery will work too, as it, like carrots, keeps in the fridge for weeks, though I personally consider organic raw celery a tad fibrous at this stage. And, of course, slap on several tablespoons of the aforementioned fermented vegetables and the stick-to-the-ribs avocados. The dried seaweed dulce I sprinkle on salads as well. It has no taste and as previously noted, is mineral-rich. And please find the courage to put some heat in that salad, as hot peppers support better health, including weight loss, help with depression, cancer prevention and heart disease prevention (40). My personal salad has few ingredients: greens, avocado, scallions and cultured veggies with homemade cayenne-infused salad dressing. Please don't let me see one more person at the salad bar slathering a bowl of nutrition with ranch

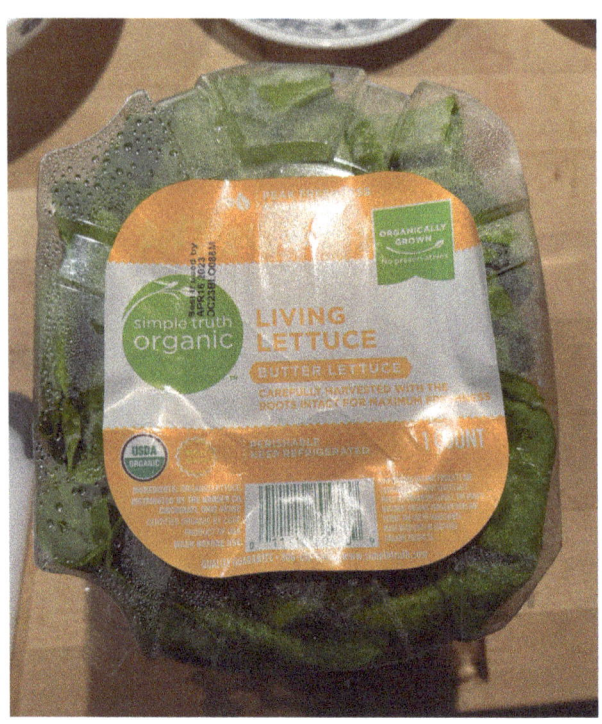

dressing and fried onions! Organic apple cider vinegar and extra virgin olive oil, both true longevity wonders, and a little cayenne tincture are all you need. Add ginger and garlic to spice it up. These foods increase inner movement through the system and decrease inflammation. (And kudos to The Egg Bistro right there in downtown Butts Station for making the dressed arugula salad a side dish option instead of the delicious yet enzyme-bereft grits or home-fried potatoes!)

Bottom line: daily salads are a big part of maintaining healthy pH in the body, which guards against cancers and other diseases. Cancer likes acidity. Let's not give it a foothold in our systems. And please consider anything that may irritate your system such as onions or peppers to omit. Also the option of eating something spicy earlier in the day may make for a better night's sleep.

SHELLED HEMP

Hemp is another very healthy food—a complete food, balanced with healthy protein, carbs and fat. It's protein is more accessible than animal protein, as it is more easily digestible. As it is also packed with minerals and amino acids, humans could, if necessary, live on shelled hemp (3). I load my morning drink with shelled hemp hearts and occasionally sprinkle them on a salad or even cereal to boast nutritional value.

As environmental issues arise, because of its availability and ease to produce, hemp could eventually replace animal meat as the world's protein source. You can purchase shelled hemp at Walmart or order it on Amazon.

BITTER FOODS

Sweet stuff tastes good; bitter stuff tastes bad. We all grew up with this knowledge, to our detriment. As a kid I only wanted to eat sweet foods. Yet have you noticed how practically all types of medicine are bitter? There has to be a common thread between bitterness and better health. Bitter foods increase pH, support food digestion and naturally detoxify the body (6). My personal favorite bitter food is, of course, aloe, then grapefruits, lemons, limes, Granny Smith apples and kiwifruit. Trader Joe's sells an unsweetened (*not* from concentrate) jar of cranberry juice, which I will occasionally pull out of the fridge and swig. Will wake you up! I also take herbal digestive bitters I purchase from the Surthrival website, which stimulates the salivary glands and releases digestive enzymes.

FERMENTED DAIRY

Fermented foods have been a part of our dietary culture since the onset of civilization. Its initial use was to prolong food availability. Benefits include colon health improvement, obesity, inflammation reduction and improved cognitive function (23). I occasionally eat yogurt. From the study "Fermented Dairy Foods: Impact on Intestinal Microbiota and Health Linked Biomarkers," *yogurt showed a higher ability to modulate the fecal microbiota*, which is kind of wordy and means it creates healthy microbes in the colon (23).

I eat no-frills low fat (dairy is a saturated fat) unsweetened yogurt and sweeten my yogurt with fruit. If you must sweeten yours further, please use honey. It's the healthiest choice.

Fermented kefir is another choice, as its liquidity makes it easier to consume. Also coconut water kefir, a *Body Ecology* discovery, is an option. It's nutritious and probiotic-packed, though take it easy with all fermented consumption at first, as it may create gas in the system.

I've written of the many impactful foods and health-related substances I've been using over the years that I believe help me continue an active, productive life. Just as I've noted the additions to my diet, now we need to address the foods and habits that need serious tweaking or removing altogether. I'm strongly of the opinion healthy nutrition for the elderly isn't so much about what to add but more about what to omit, so please take this section seriously.

FOODS AND HABITS TO TWEAK OR OMIT

SUGAR
(AND ALL PROCESSED CARBOHYDRATES)

At one time, sugar was either extremely rare or too expensive for regular folks to purchase. Not anymore. If you are in your fifties, sixties, or older, there's a high probability you have, at least to some degree, an addiction to sugar (7). Looking for a nutritional bad guy? Sugar is it, though most sweet foods now processed and consumed in America come from corn, not actual cane. In the article "Sugar Addiction: Pushing the Drug-Sugar Analogy to the Limit," we read, "Sugar…can induce…cravings that are comparable in magnitude to those induced by addictive drugs" (7). Also, in the article titled "Intense Sweetness Surpasses Cocaine Reward," the authors assert sweet foods that were absent in the human diet until very recently are clinically proven more addictive to lab rats than cocaine" (8). And what does cancer thrive on? "Preclinical studies…show that high-sucrose…diets activate several mechanistic pathways…suggesting a causal link between excess sugar consumption and cancer development…" (25).

But, honestly, folks, do I have to dig up the mountains of research that support the fact that sugar is addictive? It pervades society. And I willingly admit I am absolutely a lifelong sugar junkie. Born and raised on the stuff—soft drinks, cookies, candy and sugar-infused processed meals. And don't get me started on all the sugar-soaked cereal I ate. As a teenager, I was able to eat an entire box of Captain Crunch in one sitting—couldn't get enough. Now I have made huge strides with respect to my sugar consumption, using good fats, yogurt, kefir and cultured veggies to quell my urges. To my credit, some treats, such as candy bars, soft drinks and anything with icing on it are now simply too sweet for me to consume. Yet I must remain forever diligent to keep sugar and all processed carbs to a minimum. I cannot write strongly enough on the importance of quelling sugar consumption. It causes cancer, inflammation and obesity; it stiffens the joints, hardens the arteries and dulls the mind (14).

The current conception seemingly raised by the media and the young that it's fine to be larger and weigh more than your natural age and weight is, to me, at least questionable. I understand this is a complex issue and there are genetic and hormonal responses certain people receive with respect to their size and weight. Still, I believe it is our personal responsibility to do all we can to be healthy and not fall into nutritional misbehavior simply because it's trending. Now I don't want to attack but rather empathize with this group, to break down why we eat what we eat. To summarize Clampolini, et al, *recognizing* true hunger symptoms (stomach growling, light-headedness) as opposed to a glycemic episode (low blood sugar, body freaking out), as well as moving away from traditional consumption habits (must eat three meals a day, etc.) are key to establishing better health (73).

A while back I read a book titled *There Is a Cure for Diabetes* written by Gabriel Cousins. There was also a film based upon the book, where several people diagnosed with diabetes were taken away from their homes and unhealthy habits and fed a plant and fruit raw-food diet. The folks that toughed it out and stayed were eventually taken off their medications.

Many of my older relatives dealt with diabetes in their lifetimes. Not having to deal with it gives me the impression my diet has given me the ability to control it. Eating healthy fats, as well as consuming probiotics and enzymes with cultured veggies, yogurt and kefir works for me. Also, for many years, I have replaced sugar with Lakanto Monkfruit sweetener, zero glycemic, zero calorie, all natural. And as previously mentioned, MCT oil powder does give a degree of sweetness when added to foods.

We must also watch out for nonnutritive sweeteners like aspartame and saccharin, man-made, fake, not natural. I wouldn't eat it—neither should you.

Folks, I believe this to be the main health challenge in this stage of our lives—to control processed or really any type of carbohydrates. We must tame this beast.

CIGARETTE SMOKING

Honestly, do I have to dig up research to prove smoking cigarettes is bad for you? It's been conventional wisdom for over fifty years. And yet, whenever I work on large construction job-sites, I'm sometimes gagged by cigarette smoke. Didn't these guys get the message that smoking causes cancer? Now I know nicotine is incredibly addictive and it's very tough to quit smoking. But I have a relative who attended a no-smoking hypnosis seminar and since then, hasn't smoked a single cigarette. Quitting is possible.

Here are three consequences of smoking and some very good reasons to quit:

1. Going blind—increases the risk of age-related macular generation, also the leading cause of blindness in people over sixty-five.

2. Type two diabetes—creates poor blood flow to lower limbs. May cause infection, possibly amputation.

3. Erectile dysfunction—causes narrowing of blood vessels, including those that supply blood to the penis.

The list goes on and on, including hip fractures, colorectal cancer, rheumatoid arthritis and gum disease (37).

In the words of Dr. Richard Schulze, "You can't be a smoker and be healthy."

A while back, I was riding home from work, listening to a researcher on the radio speak about how women who smoked during pregnancy had an increased risk of their children having lower math and science scores in school. Since I've never been good at math, I wondered about this and at the next opportunity asked my mother if she smoked while I lived in her womb.

"Oh, yeah," was her response and she said it quite matter-of-factly.

I asked her why on the earth she would do that.

"The doctor told me to."

"Your doctor told you to smoke? While pregnant?"

"Yup, he told me to smoke—it would help keep my weight down."

Such was 1957 medical wisdom?

Wow…

DECREASE MEAT CONSUMPTION

In spite of the Paleo diet's claim that eating a hunter-gatherer diet is a healthy choice, it seems modern meat consumption has its drawbacks, especially processed meats containing nitrosamines, chemicals that cause cancer in laboratory animals and humans (61). "Convincing association was found between larger intake of red meat and cancer...increased consumption of processed meat was also found to be associated with colorectal, esophageal, gastric and bladder cancer" (9).

I know a fellow whose basic meat consumption is wild deer. Good for him—that's wild-harvested, natural protein, though I personally have no interest in shooting a deer or killing any animal. I guess I must be more gatherer than hunter, though I'm ruthless to mosquitoes and horseflies. But if you're eating lots of red and specifically processed meat like hotdogs or bologna, your cancer risks increase. My general rule is to eat red meat seldom, really just a few times a year. Any red meat I would consume should be high quality and pasture raised, if possible. Mostly I stick to chicken, which I consume a couple times a month on average. Wild-caught seafood is also an option, though it's rare.

It would also be wise to consume meat earlier in the day, as eating meat in the evening "may diminish sleep quality and slow digestion causing acid reflux, even high blood pressure" (42). Also, please omit grilling meat or even toasting bread to the point of blackening, as it creates two carcinogens: heterocyclic aromatic amines (HCA) and polycyclic aromatic hydrocarbons (PAH), which alter DNA wherein cancers may form (52).

EASY ON THE BOOZE

I have several friends who, after reading this heading, will be driving over to slug me for suggesting they cut back on their favorite beer. But most types of beer contain gluten and as suggested in *The Plant Paradox*, gluten is a lectin, which creates havoc in the bowels, the immune system and general health. Dr. Gundry suggests red wine or dark whiskey as an alternative. There are also gluten-free beers to purchase. Dark beer contains more gluten than light beer (68). Common sense suggests smaller portions as we age.

Alcohol consumption was a very big part of my younger adult life. Change is difficult but necessary as we age. In the last few years I've cut way back on alcohol as it now irritates my system; too much stiffens joints, creates an erratic sleep pattern and over time may raise my blood pressure (44). Alcohol isn't a type of food and is not digested like food. It's broken down in the liver, which responds to it as a toxin and must work hard to remove it. It has no nutritional value and inhibits essential mineral absorption (60). Also "heavy drinking can be a leading cause of candida (yeast) overgrowth…" (26). And any type of alcohol dehydrates the system. Studies show that for every alcoholic drink you drink, your body must expel four times as much liquid (51). This can be dangerous for the elderly. We must take the possibility of dehydration seriously. And we must make a tough decision.

Folks, if our essential goal is optimum health and alcohol consumption detracts from this goal, the only choice is to either abstain or cut way back on its use. Anyone diagnosed with an illness should seriously consider giving up all alcohol consumption.

PLEASE CONSIDER RED WINE

Red wine contains the phenol (pigment) resveratrol, which explains the French paradox: why the French can indulge in rich foods yet are not plagued with American diseases. Resveratrol promotes healthy gut function, reduces inflammation and supports cardio function (22). Also, red wine isn't gassy. Beer *is* gassy and nutritionally doesn't promote better health. And as per the last section, please go easy on alcohol consumption, if not completely abstaining.

WOMEN WITH BREAST IMPLANTS— ANOTHER TOUGH DECISION!

Ladies, ask any of my male friends, there's no bigger fan than myself, but as of October 2021, "Breast implants have been linked to cancer of the immune system and a host of other medical conditions including autoimmune diseases, joint pain, mental confusion, muscle aches and chronic fatigue" (12).

No one hates to see them go more, but your white blood cells are needed elsewhere. Breast implants are foreign entities to which your immune system must respond. My friends with hip or knee replacements tell me they take prescribed drugs to fight off their immune system's response. It was probably okay in your youth to have breast implants when you had a young, strong immune system. At this stage, we must do all we can to keep our systems strong.

AND SPEAKING OF HIP/KNEE REPLACEMENTS

Though it sounds medieval, having a surgeon open you up and hammering a fake bone part inside of you, I have heard positive results do come from this procedure. And it wouldn't surprise me if, because of my own sports-related bone-loss issues, a replacement of some type could be in my future, though I will do all I can to prevent it. But to all who are thinking of getting any kind of bone, joint, hip or knee replacement, please consider some sort of weight-loss program first. It may be all you need.

GIVE UP CAFFEINE

Little known fact: older adults drink more coffee than any other age group. And although caffeine is an antioxidant, it is also classified as a drug and may create such risks as stress on the kidneys and bladder and elevated blood pressure. Caffeine also, like alcohol, dehydrates to a degree (13).

I have two friends with heart concerns who were advised by their doctors not to consume drinks containing caffeine. I do not drink caffeinated coffee, nor have I consumed a soft drink in this century, so it won't trouble me personally. It just makes sense to me for older people not to jolt themselves out of morning sluggishness with a hit from a drug called caffeine.

Just saying…

HEALTHY HABITS TO TRY/CONSIDER

PEACE OF MIND

Research shows that optimism's positive effects are associated with better health (22). All right, positive emotions create better health and longevity. Easy to say, tough to do when you're driving down the road, heading home, about to enter the tunnel when a wrecker truck crosses the solid line right in front of you and simultaneously shoots a rock into your windshield.

Actually happened not long ago.

The point here is it's very difficult not to become occasionally upset unless you're living in a Buddhist temple somewhere in Tibet. Stuff happens and we get mad. That's bad for the elderly. Our aging cardiovascular systems do not need stress. The puzzlement of new technologies, as well as confounding social trends don't help either. Reading Eckhart Tolle's *The Power of Now* has been helpful to quell my occasional pessimism. *A Course in Miracles*, which I have been reading for many years and define as a new age foundation of the Christian faith, has made a difference. Stripping judgment and guilt from our minds brings peace; this book has been helpful in that process. Also Daniel Goleman's *Emotional Intelligence* helped clarify many erratic and impulsive tendencies.

Depression is a common issue for geezers. Many are lonely and isolated. Many have, over the years, picked up terrible dietary habits. But in *Foods that Help Battle Depression*, the author writes of a study of sixty-seven people suffering depression, half given social support and half given nutritional counseling. After twelve weeks, the people who improved their diets showed significantly happier moods than those who received social support. And the people who improved their diets the most improved the most (31).

Guilt and shame are two emotions that slowly strip us of health and well-being. They can lead to depression, anxiety and paranoia, yet, when we are honest and not withholding truth, may move us back to peace (34). It's never too late to clean up perceived emotional failures if we find the courage to do so. Perhaps all of us have, to a degree, emotional memories that sap us of inner peace. Never too late to clean this up with a meeting, even a phone call.

Peace of mind is worth more than any possession. Create a diet that uplifts you. Find inspiration wherever you can. If your job brings you down, get a new one. If you're around pessimism, move away. If someone pulls energy from you, run.

We have been alive a long time. It hasn't been easy. Acknowledge the strength it took to get this far.

ORTHOTICS

Twenty or so years ago, I made the bad decision to play old boys rugby. I had played as a young man (was never tough but always quick) and thought it would be fun to relive the excitement. I originally stopped playing in my youth, as my left shoulder kept popping out at practice. But that was many years ago and said shoulder hadn't given me problems, though I wasn't immune to receiving new injuries. There's the previously mentioned Boulder lower back injury of 2015 in Aspen, as well as the Mystic River right shoulder injury of 2017 at Saranac Lake.

But the last year or so, I've been feeling a new symptom with my hips, a sharp pain in one or the other. And as I refuse to go under the knife, I sought an alternative, which led me to The Good Feet Store in Hilltop. I had seen several commercials about the store and heard testimonials from folks swearing this stuff works, so I bought in.

After being set up with correct orthotics, the first thing I noticed when I stood up was how amazingly level I felt. I really had no idea how out-of-whack my bones were. I obviously had an improper foundation, which I blame on wearing an out-of-balance tool belt for so many years. The system takes several weeks, using different types of orthotics, but never completely ends as we must adjust to aging and its toils.

I will continue to use this system as long as it works for me. I'm also swearing off my tool belt, which seems impossible to balance and has been creating compression on my hips for many years. I also bought a pair of orthotic-type flip-flops from the store, far superior to any flip-flop I've ever worn. Its soft foam cushion really allows for a hugged-foot experience; does not slide around on your feet like other types of flip-flops.

HAVE YOUR DNA TESTED

My results from 23andMe from January 2024 are as follows:

99.7 percent European…of which I'm…
38.7 percent French/German
36.6 percent Irish/English
9.4 percent Broadly Southern European
And a few trace percentages…

I'm also related way down the line to Marie Antoinette and Niall, an ancient Irish king. Though interesting, what I needed to learn was my genetic predisposition to illness. What I've got isn't terrible, but good to know, as perhaps my diet will help quell possible affliction. Three notifications came up:

Looks like I have an AAT deficiency that may lead to lung and liver disease, though it's considered *not likely at risk*. I have one of two genetic variants for celiac disease, though according to my last colonoscopy, my colon is in very healthy shape. Alas, the last, for age-related macular degeneration, I have *both* genetic markers. I need to keep an eye (no pun intended) on this particular genetic weakness. And as part of my health protocol, I've added the keto-carotenoid astaxanthin, which is not only known to improve eye health (54) but also to improve, according to a friend, libido, a topic I'd rather not open, though perhaps I should.

LIBIDO—OKAY, HERE GOES...

Honestly, do our bodily urges serve us with respect to the understanding and nature of actual love? Lust isn't love; it's a powerful hormonal urge. And this notion of wanting to strengthen sex drive with a libido-enhancing pill at an elderly age, to me seems risky. Health issues such as low blood pressure, sickle cell anemia, heart attack and stroke have me thinking we should leave such products alone (48).

EARTHING

Did you know the earth we exist on is like a giant electron battery, that its core, along with the thousands of lightning strikes it absorbs every day creates enormous health benefits? And did you know we humans don't receive those benefits because we insulate ourselves with rubber-soled shoes? That's basically the premise of "Earthing," published in 2014, which scientifically proves "grounding" yourself, simply walking barefoot on the ground, will reunite you with the natural electrical systems of the earth. Our bodies are electrically (and chemically) run. When we "earth," we become grounded and in so doing receive negatively charged electrons naturally rising from the ground, eliminating excess free radicals and creating a more smoothly run system. The electron absorption also reduces inflammation, the cause of many health issues, including arrythmias, autism, diabetes and cancer. "Earthing" greatly reduces the effects of EMFs on the human system. It even helps deal with emotional issues as it lifts the spirits (24). "The biological clock of the body needs to be continually calibrated by the pulse of the earth that governs the circadian rhythms of all life on the planet" (24).

So are you ready to give up those rubber-soled shoes in the dead of winter? Not necessary! There are lots of "grounding" products available to purchase online: sheets, blankets, shoes and mats to put your feet on while you work. I have a "grounding" pillowcase. It's inexpensive, effective and connects to the part of my body needing the most attention. I have found my sleeping is much deeper on my "earthed" pillow.

More on sleep needs later…

ENEMAS

"The colon is the second brain," writes Dr. Gundry. Our mouths are only the sweet end of approximately thirty feet of digestive track. By the time what we ate gets to the other end, our bodies have not only dealt with digested food but also discarded toxic cellular waste. Combine that with the less-than-healthy standard foods consumed, a colon flushing seems reasonable to me. Humans have been taking enemas since the days of ancient Egypt, possibly longer (10). I've read the pros and cons concerning whether or not they are healthy, but I began doing enemas about twenty years ago via the advice of a holistic health counselor who was a strong advocate. High enemas are also part of Dr. Schulze's *Incurables Program*. Is doing an enema fun? Not really, but it isn't painful, just a tad awkward. Like so many of the practices I do for better health, I do enemas because I believe they are good for me. It's like getting your car's oil changed. It makes sense to have the engine's inner walls occasionally flushed.

How do you do an enema? I'll give it a shot. Put a quart of filtered, warm water in an enema bag, lie on your back (I do mine on the floor on a towel, though most older folks should be elevated), rub a little coconut oil on the tube, insert the tube in your you-know-where and pop the shut-off snapper to allow the water to flow. Press the snapper in to slow the flow of water if it feels uncomfortable. When it's time to release the water from your colon and into the toilet, you'll know. And on a personal note, please *do not* leave the bathroom while holding the liquid in your colon. You never know when you have to release it into the toilet.

Folks, I understand there may be an aversion to performing this procedure on yourself, but in March of 2023, I had my second colonoscopy, not fun, but was thrilled to learn by the performing doctor my colon was in "very healthy" shape: no polyps, masses or diverticulitis.

DETOXIFICATION

As important as consuming healthy foods is ridding your body of waste. Here's a quote from Richard Schulze, a doctor of holistic medicine in practice for over forty years:

> Every one of the 37 trillion cells in your body creates metabolic waste as it functions…Every cell relies on your body's garbage disposal systems—your bowel, liver and kidneys—to remove waste from your body. When any of these waste disposal systems gets congested, cellular waste backs up. This is a serious problem…Routine seasonal detoxification is preventative maintenance for your body (64).

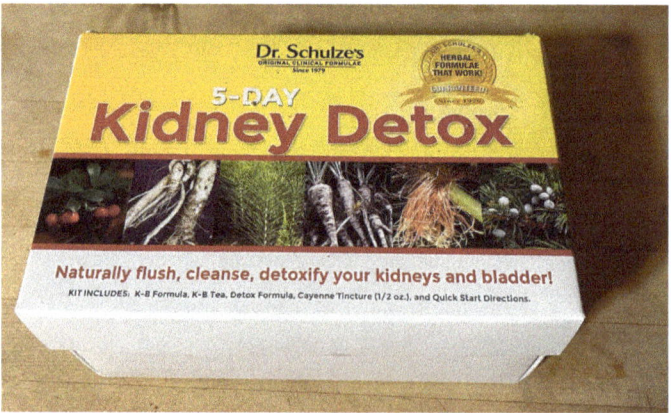

Compound cellular waste with the 188 toxic air pollutants in the air we breathe, the water we drink, the outdoors and in our homes, detoxification is crucial (39). Dr. Schulze recommends detoxifying with the change of seasons, four times a year. I've been practicing this for at least fifteen years—for kidneys, liver, and colon, our basic detoxification organs. How extreme you're willing to go depends on how well you want the detox to work, as well as your personal fortitude. I have done all juice detoxes; my favorite is cucumber, apple, lime and ginger, though I would need to stay home to do this type. Since I still need to work, I usually do a raw food detox. As long as I have avocados, it's not a problem. Also, when we detoxify, we release acidity from our system (4).

I start every morning doing a simple detox. Detoxification methods include *oil pulling* (swishing coconut oil in your mouth) while I simultaneously perform *dry brushing* (brushing my entire body with a stiff brush). Both stimulate the lymphatic system. I brush around my groin, armpit and neck areas mostly, as that's where our lymph nodes concentrate. I also drink warm lemon water and then a shot of apple cider vinegar. This takes only a few minutes. Oil pulling has another attribute: coconut oil naturally whitens teeth! Also, I occasionally drink a bentonite clay and water concoction (Intestinal #2) to clean out my intestines, which promotes mineral absorption (36).

Folks, please take this aspect of health seriously. Take the time, spend the money.

You must detox!!!

PURE WATER

Is your tap water safe to drink? If you want to know, visit the ewg.org tap water database to find out. The city I live in provides water analysis on their website. And though it seems I have *safe* water coming out of my faucet, it has a swampy ditch smell and tastes similar, so I purchased a Propur three-gallon gravity-driven system. The filters are a tad on the expensive side but last several years. Also, please consider ordering a lemon wedge with water at restaurants, helps disinfect…

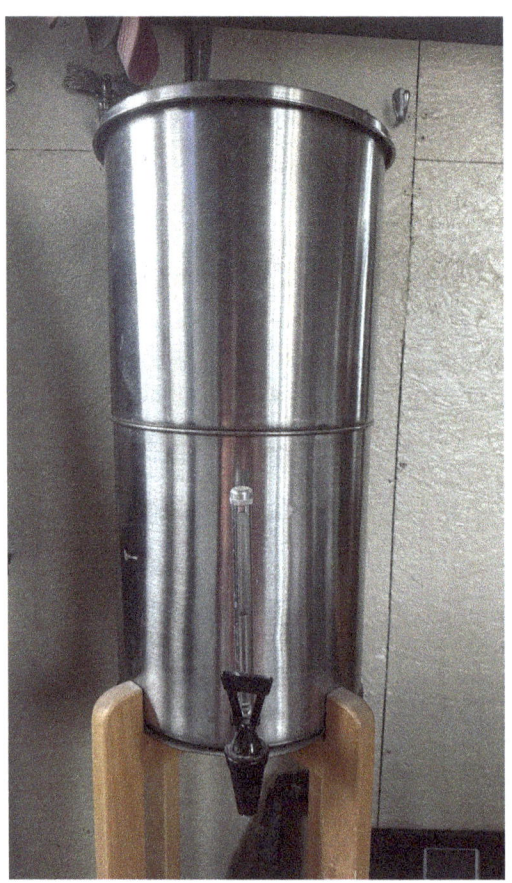

IMPORTANCE OF CONSUMING ORGANIC

I've read that organic fruits and vegetables are healthier for us than the regular type, and I've read there's no difference. Whatever the standards, I choose to purchase organic food whenever possible because they aren't sprayed with the evil herbicide Roundup, as its residuals on food wreak havoc in the bowels (6). Since GMOs were basically designed to work with Roundup, seems to me that we should leave genetically modified foods alone whenever possible. Organic food is available at Trader Joe's and Walmart.

Old folks are more vulnerable to chemicals and I know we can't always, but whenever possible, choose organic!

READ INGREDIENTS AND NUTRITIONAL FACTS LABELS

I can and occasionally do spend hours in the grocery store reading the labels of food I'm thinking of purchasing. I figure it's my responsibility to know what's in any food before I consume it. We need to check the ingredients. For example, I really loved Cheetos in my youth but don't eat them anymore because the oil used to make them is either corn, canola, and/or sunflower. The last oil, sunflower, I don't mind. The other two I don't want in my body. Trader Joe's sells a Cheeto alternative, Fancy Cheese Crunchies, that contains only sunflower oil, healthier because of it's stability (69). They don't have the crunch of the original Cheetos but are healthier because of the oil used to create them.

We also have to be careful with how clever, yet insidious, food manufacturers can be. Watch the *number of servings* or *portions per package* with respect to *fat* content and *sugar* content. A label can read *one gram of fat per serving* and also read *five servings* in the *Nutritional Facts* block. We must watch the number of different types of sugar on the label: corn syrup, tapioca and so on. And watch out for types of *sugar alcohols* instead of sugar. We must also be very careful with respect to buzz words on the front of the package that fool you into purchasing the item even though the food label gives you a different story. The wording on the front of the package isn't always governed by law (61).

Watch the *Ingredients* and *Nutritional Facts* labels like a hawk!

COOK WITH NONVOLATILE SURFACES

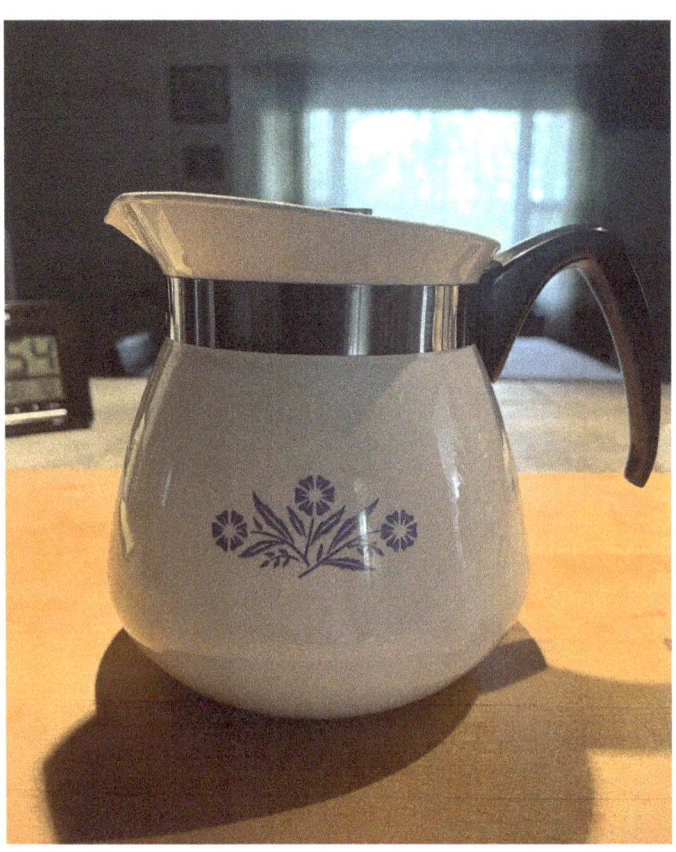

My mom, early on, used big cast iron cookware to cook our meals. Sometime in the early seventies, she, being a *modern lady*, switched to Teflon cookware, which may be another explanation as to why I'm terrible at math. Turns out Teflon contains perfluorooctanoic acid, which disrupts lots of human body processes (29). Nowadays pots and pans are safer, though good old cast iron is safe (70) as its composition doesn't leach into food. I have also used ceramic cookware sold on the Dr. Mercola website. And my mother's eighties Corning Ware works great and is considered stable (71).

AVOID CHEMICALS

I use Tom's of Maine deodorant as after researching, I found its ingredients are basically benign. I brush with Burt's Bees charcoal toothpaste, though folks on prescribed medications may wish to abstain because of possible side-effects of charcoal. Removing food and plaque is important, as the bacteria in plaque creates an acidic condition in the mouth, which in time breaks down tooth enamel (49).

I have found, at this stage, any type soap dries my skin. As an alternative I wash with warm water and lemon juice. I feel clean, it doesn't leave me feeling crusty, and I need not wash it off. I use coconut oil as a moisturizer and an antibacterial. As a rule, I brush, floss, *and* gargle at least once every day, usually twice if possible. Flossing is very important, as it aids in removing harmful bacteria from your mouth (72). Considering our bacteria-laden mouths are just a few inches from our brains, it is an obvious necessity to keep teeth clean. Gargling is also important, as it is a kind of pressure washing of the mouth and is especially

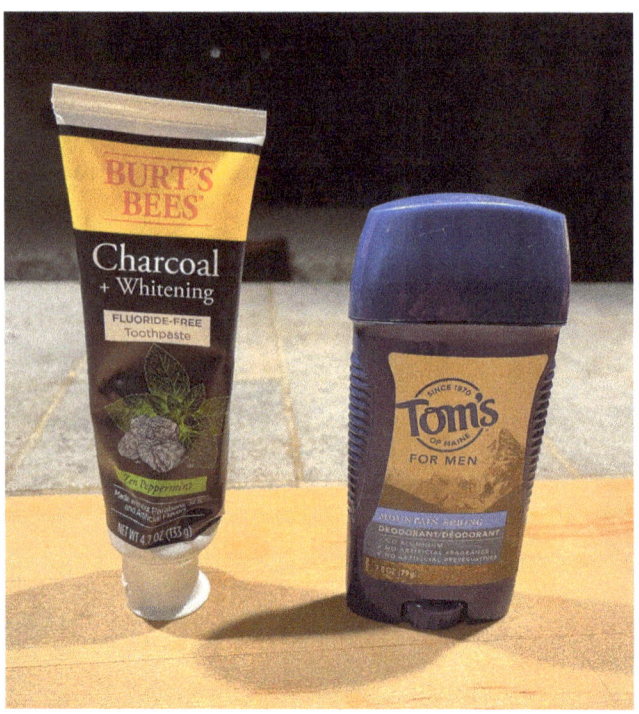

important in the morning for obvious reasons. I use lemon juice to wash dishes. I wash clothes free of perfumes, dyes, anything that irritates skin. I clean my house with Trader Joe's cedar wood and sage cleaner.

For immediate pain relief, I take aspirin internally, Biofreeze externally, and aloe both ways. Take it easy with aspirin, as it may irritate the stomach lining (6).

SEE A CHIROPRACTOR REGULARLY

Getting a chiropractic adjustment gives positive effects to the human body. It works on inflammation, flexibility, blood flow and pressure, digestion, sleep and even vertigo (47).

I've been seeing chiropractors for at least thirty-five years. For me personally, chiropractic adjustments improve any pain or discomfort I'm feeling at any specific time. Headaches have been an ongoing health concern for me since childhood, though I believe now it was mostly a symptom of an awful diet. Age is probably the reason now. When I see a chiropractor, it's almost always because of neck soreness and stiffness and my now perpetual lower-back sports injury. And my most recent chiropractor is full contact! This fellow does not mess around. I feel much looser and relaxed after the visit.

On April 2, 2024, I went in for an adjustment. The chiropractor asked me if I was careful with the food I ate. When I told him yes, he responded he was not surprised, as I was very easy to adjust as there seemed a lack of inflammation in my joints for a fellow my age.

Something to consider…

MOVEMENT

I once read how the two greatest aspects of health and longevity were calorie restriction and physical activity. People living in vast, isolated regions with no televisions or cell phones, who work from sun-up to sun-down creating food, are the healthiest people on the planet. Dr. Jensen, in his book, *Guide to Body Chemistry and Nutrition*, wrote of how the Hunza Valley people of Pakistan thrived in this way, secluded high in the mountains, drinking mineral-rich glacial water. Some lived up to 140 years.

The diet I suggest in this book I believe will take care of calorie restriction. We all need to figure out a way to move. My occupation handles that for the most part: I build things—physically. I do tai chi form practice. You may have seen folks moving very slowly in the park, moving arms, slowly turning. That's tai chi form, nothing abrupt or jerky. I take my dog for walks in the park or on the beach. I surf in the summer when the water is warm and there are casual-size waves. Riding a bike could be a better option for some as it's easier on the joints. But honestly, I don't do much physically anymore on Sundays. I use them to relax and recuperate. I move plenty during the week, though.

You do what you need to do to get moving. Join a gym like East Coast Gym in Virginia Beach (I hear it's great!). There are tai chi and yoga classes, or you can just take a walk in your neighborhood. And before you do anything, create a stretch protocol for yourself. I begin stretching before I get out of bed and continue, standing, first thing every morning!

News Flash! From February 26, 2024, from local Channel 13 news…to paraphrase, persons with sedentary workplace conditions or lackadaisical lifestyles in general are linked to potential health risks such as diabetes, chronic inflammation, hypertension, osteoporosis, depression, cancer and cognitive impairment. This was backed up with research (55).

GET A DOG

Dogs in your life boost your quality of life. They lower blood pressure and cholesterol, reduce the risk of heart attack and help with human interaction (32).

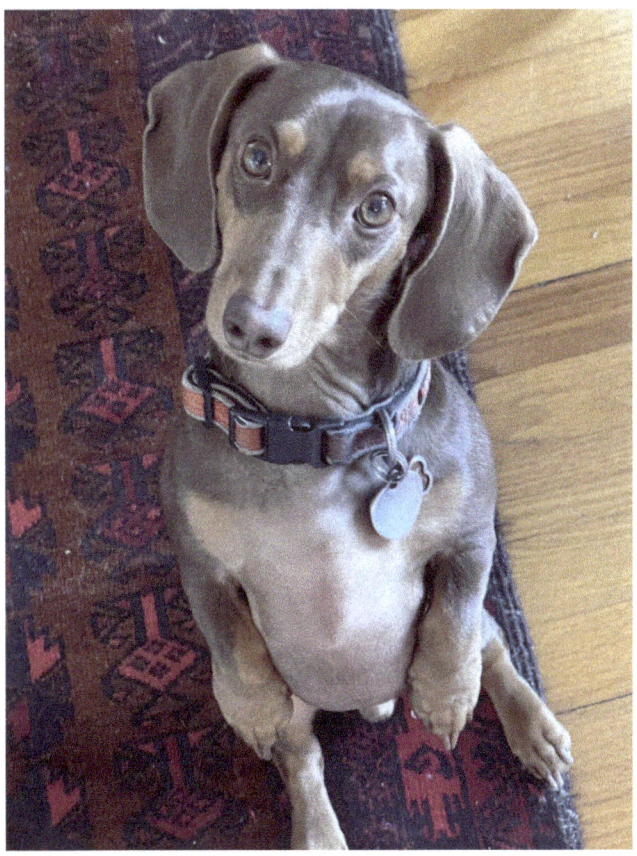

I live with a stubborn, cover-stealing, snuggling-till-I-get-pushed-off-the-bed wiener dog and I wouldn't have it any other way. He is a noble creature, both clever and brave, and stands between me and anything that would harm me. He eats food of the highest quality; his bowl is washed after every meal. He gnaws on yak cheese chews as they are the safest. He deserves to be pampered.

RAISE YOUR TELEVISION SET

My Facebook page constantly reminds me of something I already know, which is how sore and tender my neck has become over the years. There are posts showing all sorts of medieval-type products for stretching the neck and relieving pain caused by the constant bending of our necks downward, pretty much from anything that directs our interest toward our phones. Pain is caused by nerve compression, old sports injuries and the straining of muscles, to name a few (50). Some preventions include raising the height of your phone so you aren't constantly looking down. Thinking how often we watch television, it makes sense to me to install a TV hanger high up on a wall or even attached to the ceiling, which would raise the television up high in the room and create less stress on our necks. I'm pretty much a sports and movie watcher, though if there's a *Game of Thrones* marathon on, I can't help but at least tune in during commercials.

STORE FOOD IN GLASS AND STAINLESS STEEL BEFORE PLASTIC

Dr. Gundry recommends avoiding plastics as much as possible. Compounds such as BPA and phthalates found in plastic bags, rubber gloves and so on may be toxic to the human system (6). According to the box, the Ziploc-brand plastic bags are BPA-free. With respect to plastics, always seek BPA-free products. Stainless steel also works, though glass is the best choice—the darker the glass, the better.

GET RID OF TIGHT SOCKS

Geezers need to stay away from any clothing that may hinder circulation. So many socks, like the hiking type I once owned, are now too tight, especially around the calf area. Blood circulation to your feet is important (15). For several years, I've been wearing Dr. Scholl's Advanced Relief Casual Crew Socks I purchase at Walmart. They stay on my calves but not too tight and are cushioned on the bottom. Very comfy…

DON'T WATCH SPORTS ON TV LATE AT NIGHT

This is from Harvard Health Publishing: to paraphrase, blood pressure and heart rates rise dramatically when watching sports, especially after the team you're rooting for loses. This can have serious health consequences, such as heart failure and stroke (43). No good for Geezers…

I think it was the 2021 NCAA basketball final when the Carolina Tarheels played the Kansas Jayhawks. As a lifelong ACC fan, I rooted greatly for Carolina to win and loved the first half of the game, as Carolina was up by fifteen at the end of said half. During the intermission, I pondered whether it would be a healthy choice to stay up for the rest of the game, as a Carolina defeat would have led to me throwing things at the television and the possibility of dire conniption. I turned off the television and went to bed. Sure enough, Kansas came back and won the game, and my choice of not watching the rest of the game may have saved me from serious harm.

HAVE MERCURY REMOVED FROM YOUR MOUTH

All amalgam silver fillings contain around 50 percent mercury, a highly toxic element that has no known safe exposure level. So why is mercury used to fill teeth cavities? It's cheaper than gold, the first choice. But gold eventually became too precious, so mercury became the go-to. Also, mercury is more user-friendly and is easier to set in teeth. But some studies assert that mercury fillings may cause such health problems as headaches, kidney disease and even brain damage (16). At the advice of a holistic health counselor, I took a six-to-eight-year sojourn to have all of the mercury removed from my mouth. My insurance didn't cover dental, so I had to pay out-of-pocket each time I went to the dentist. I had each mercury filling replaced with a composite filling. Not every dentist is properly equipped for removing mercury. There are special respiratory devices both patient and dentist must wear to protect against mercury exposure. Did having the mercury removed create better health for me? I'm not sure if it did, but it's comforting to know it's gone.

EAT SOURDOUGH BREAD

If you're going to eat bread, by far and away the healthiest choice is sourdough bread. Because the dough has been fermented, the gluten in sourdough has been broken down into amino acids, making it easier to consume and digest without disturbing the colon. The type of bacteria (lactobacillus) used to ferment the dough has a beneficial effect on the system (19). It also reduces yeast, the main premise of *The Body Ecology Diet*. Trader Joe's sells excellent sourdough at a fair price. Sourdough usually comes in big slices. One piece of toast is all I need, though it's necessary to cut it in half to fit in the toaster. I usually drizzle olive or avocado oil on mine instead of butter.

WEAR COTTON CLOTHING

Cotton is natural, breathable and gentle on the skin. It absorbs moisture and doesn't trap bad smells. Polyester, though stronger and more flexible, unfortunately traps air flow next to the skin, and "IS" made of chemicals (PFCs) that absorb into the body. It also traps bad smells (20).

ENZYME SUPPLEMENTS

Our bodies are run by enzymes. There are thousands of different types: saliva enzymes, pancreatic enzymes, specific enzymes for every organ in the human body to repair damage and heal disease. The human body creates enzymes. They do a great job of this in our youth. The problem is that as we age, enzymes can and do wear out. The older we become, the less of these enzymes our bodies make. So we need to supplement what we can no longer create. One way this is done is by ***eating more raw food and less cooked food!*** "The human race is at least half sick. In a biological sense, there are no completely healthy people living on a conventional diet" (17).

Raw foods come with their own enzymes. But if your diet is mostly composed of cooked food, you should take digestive supplements. There are also foods you can create, such as the

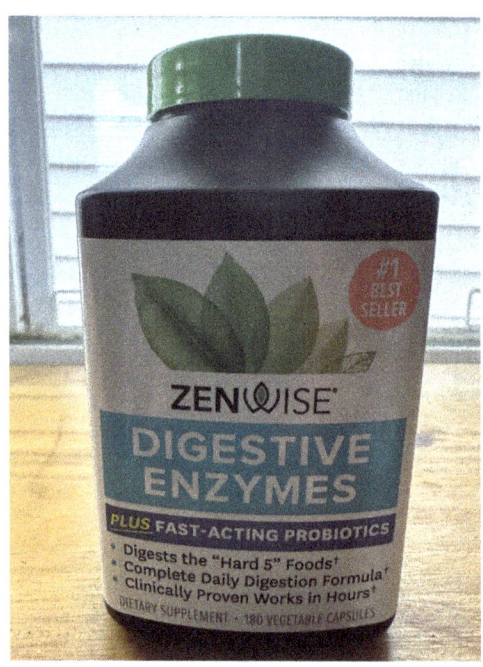

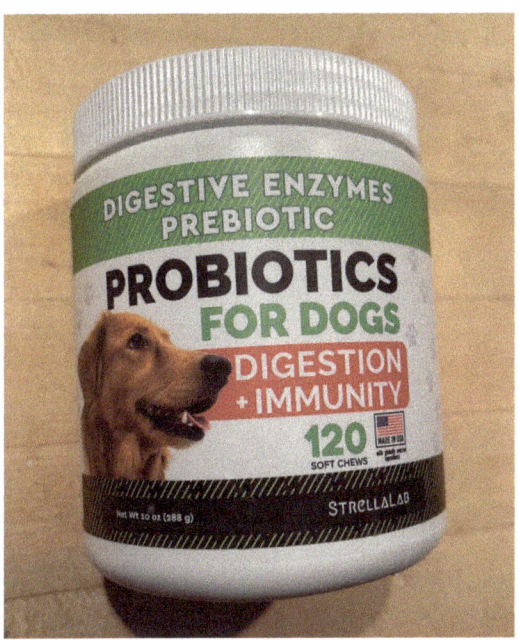

aforementioned cultured vegetables, that are packed with enzymes. A day rarely goes by without my consuming cultured vegetables. The internet is loaded with cultured vegetable recipes and tutorials. Super easy or I wouldn't be doing it.

Do you love your dog? Give him an enzyme supplement as well. They come in chewable bites sold on Amazon.

EASY ON THE SALT

I remember shaking salt all over my food in my youth. But running salt through your system strains the kidneys and circulatory system (15). Now we do need sodium intake, as it is a necessary mineral/electrolyte. It just makes sense to use it sparingly. And please purchase a quality type, such as the Himalayan Pink from Trader Joe's.

VEGANS DON'T GET CANCER

Actually, they do get cancer, but vegans, folks who "eat nothing with a face," have the lowest rate of cancer of any diet.

Vegans eat only plants or plant-based foods. Plant-based foods are composed of "phytochemicals," which are compounds that decrease inflammation and interrupt processes that encourage cancer production (27). This diet is also high in fiber, which is shown to lower cancer risks. Antioxidants and carotenoids are two types of phytochemicals.

I am still an omnivore, though through many years of trial and error and experimenting with many different methods of food consumption, I seem to have achieved a better-than-ordinary degree of health for my age. That written, the older I get, the more vegan I become.

MOVE TOWARD FRUITS

Avocados, green bananas, green apples, grapefruit and all the berries! Fruits are ready to eat, no cooking needed and stocked with vitamins, bioflavonoids, fiber and enzymes. Easy on fruits like oranges (*sweet!*) and bananas, though green bananas are fine. The brown ones are way too sweet. Please consider staying away from fruit juice, as consuming a condensed version of fruit is way too much sugar. Also please consider how eating fruits along with other types of food may create gas in the system and if so, choose to eat fruit by itself.

As much as I love berries, I suggest to all that if you're going to eat them, choose organic, as regular berries may have been chemically sprayed.

PROOF'S IN THE POOP

I believe it was Dr. Schulze who wrote how one could tell the degree of one's health by the color and density of their bowel movements. Seems a lighter, creamier movement suggests a better diet. From my experience with food choice, it's true. To make my bathroom visit more functional, I use a device I call *the poop stoop*. No, I'm not going to mass-produce them (though I could), I merely introduce a product made by others that I have used for years. It's a small step that fits in front of the toilet. The idea is to put your feet on the step, as this position mimics squatting, or how humans pooped throughout prehistory, before toilets, chamber pots, and so on. There are different styles and configurations: StrongTek, Squatty Potty, and Tushy, just to name a few.

Elimination is crucial!

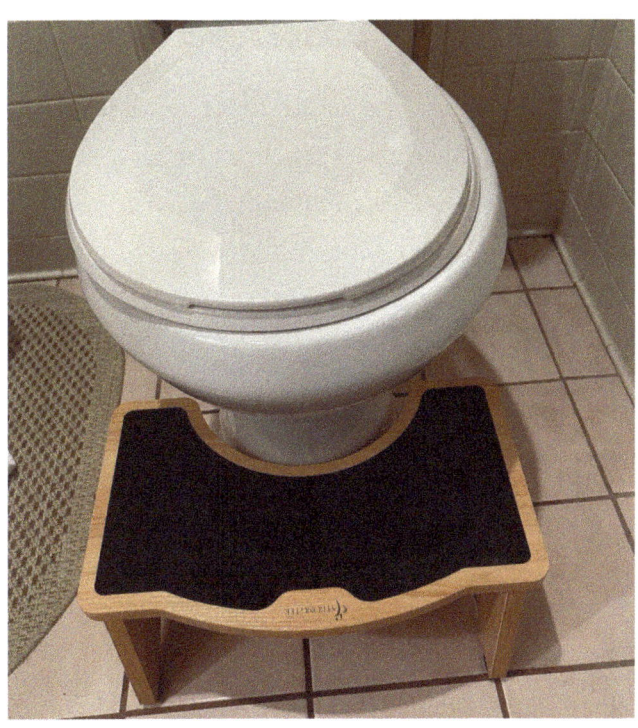

TA-65

An interesting aside: a while back, I read a book titled *The Immortality Edge*, based upon the Nobel Prize-winning research on how the shortening of chromosomal telomeres is the reason we age. Telomeres are DNA sequences at the ends of chromosomes. As cells divide over time, telomeres shorten. What bloomed from this research is a product called TA-65, which is itself an enzyme called telomerase. It's obtained from the astragalus plant, a far eastern herb. Telomerase feeds telomeres, allows them to grow longer and slows the shortening process. Could this be a serious breakthrough in the possibilities of human longevity? In 2007, after five years of research and safety testing…"A double-blind, placebo-controlled study of nearly one hundred people showed that TA-65MD significantly lengthened critically short telomeres with no serious adverse effects" (53).

With respect to the writing and research of this book, I've taken TA-65 for the last few months. It seems to have reduced joint soreness, especially my old sports injuries. The bad news is a month's supply costs six hundred bucks, out of my league at this point, though I aspire to its affordability.

TURN THE PAGE!!!

In Dr. Schulze's *20 Steps to a Healthier Life*, step number 13 reads, "Throw Away, Give Away 1/3 of Everything You Own." I understand how difficult this would be for old folks. We've spent a lifetime accumulating things that are now nostalgic and we don't want to give them up. But in the summer of '23, after many years

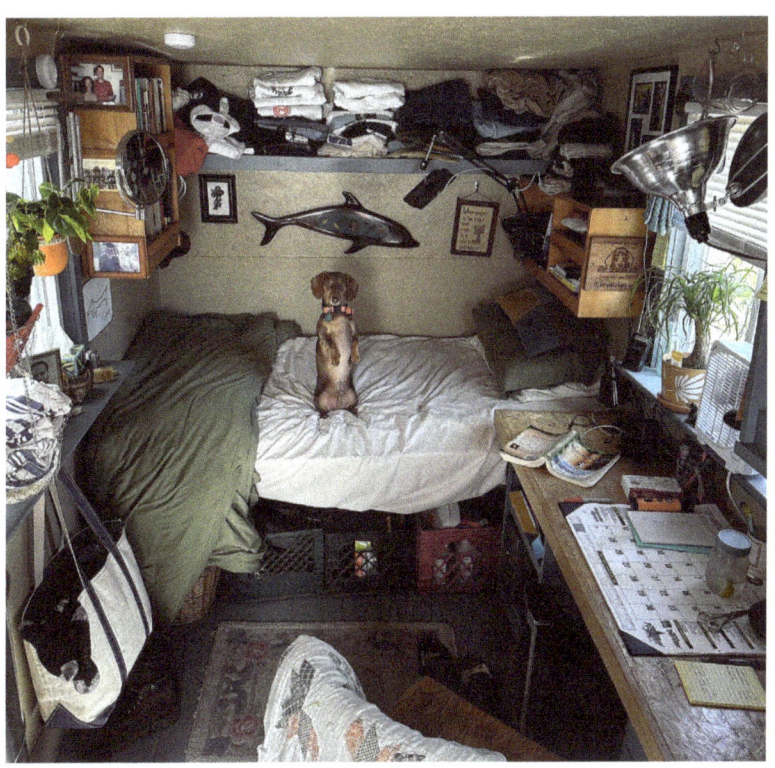

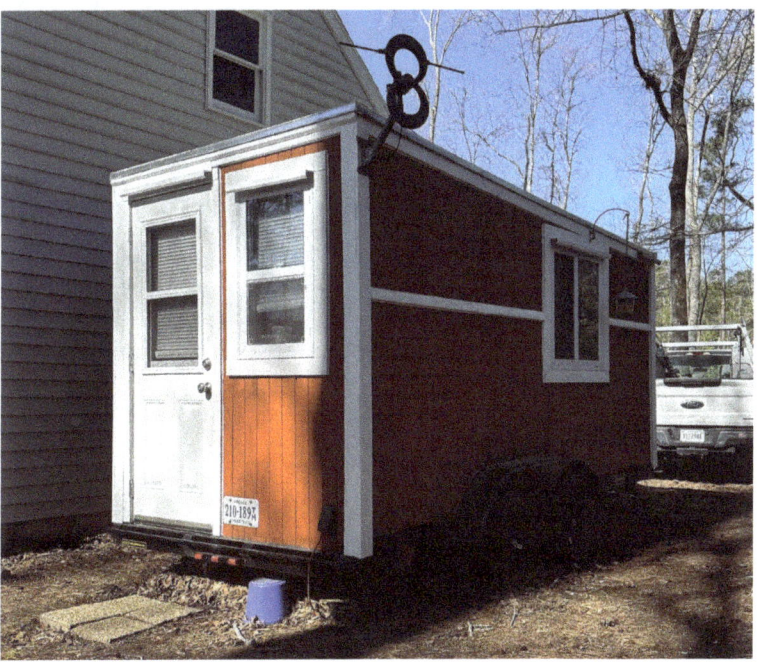

of my living in my ancestral home alone and basically living in only a few of the rooms, we decided to rent out the house while I, forgoing my plans of going broke by purchasing an Airstream travel trailer, built my own home on wheels—small but fine for one old guy and a fifteen pound wiener dog. And although leaving the home I was comfortable living in, as well as removing sixty years of most of the objects contained in said home and the emotional attachment our family had to these things, I must admit my life is now much simpler and less stressful.

NEED TO SLEEP

In his book, *The Promise of Sleep*, sleep research pioneer William Dement asserts so many of our health concerns are the effects of lack of adequate sleep. He introduces the circadian rhythms, our ancient biological clocks, which determine sleep stages, cellular activity and our need to rest in accordance with this rhythm (58). With respect to the elderly, Dement writes, "There is no question that sleep gets lighter and more fragmented as we age. Falling asleep and staying asleep are more difficult."

With respect to sleep and longevity, Dement writes, "Sleep is the most important predictor of how long you will live." Eight hours is the best amount for a night's sleep. Sleeping more or less presents problems. Compared to good sleepers, male poor sleepers were 6.5 times more likely to have health problems, and female poor sleepers were 3.5 times more likely to have health problems (58).

Sleep is also very important with respect to bodily repair, as it is during deep sleep that the process of cellular repair occurs.

Hormones, immune chemistry, the metabolic machinery, and sleep are all tied together in a complex web of biochemical interaction. Our bodies oscillate between the needs of waking life—to work, to use energy, to expose our body to wear and tear—and the necessities of renewal, when energy is stored, tissue repaired, and the immune system prepared to fight another day. (58)

Considering my personal sleep needs, my body wants to go to sleep between 8:00 and 9:00 p.m. and wake between 4:00 and 5:00 a.m. I will sometimes wake in the middle of the night and have difficulty falling back to sleep. At these times, I will read my mind-boggling chemistry book, and after about five minutes, I become drowsy. Works every time!

MORNING PROTOCOL

1. Stretch.

2. Drink one pint warm water—bite lemon wedge, then a shot of apple cider vinegar.

3. Coconut oil swish and dry brush.

4. Aloe—consume and apply to skin.

5. The morning drink.

THE MORNING DRINK

Mornings, I take many of the foods I have described in the book and make a morning drink. You may wonder if I will keep my morning mixture recipe a secret and will attempt to sell it to you for fifty bucks a jar. Nope, the ingredients in my morning drink are described in the "Foods to Add" section of the book. It is necessary for anyone reading this book to limit your consumption to small amounts of each of these ingredients first to detect any reaction you may have to each ingredient.

Morning Drink Ingredients and How to Purchase

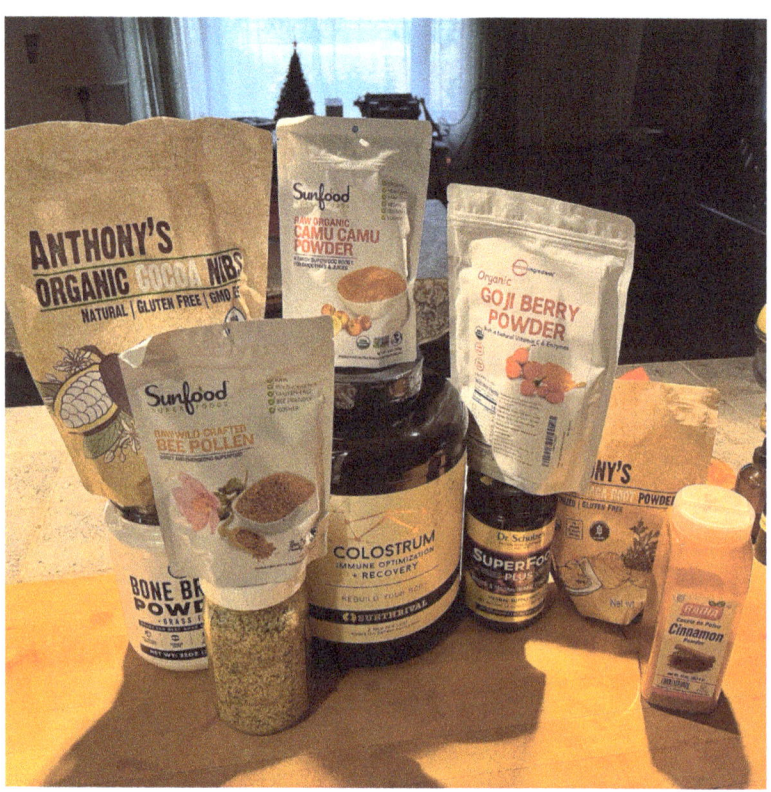

Colostrum: surthrival.com

Bone broth protein powder: leftcoastperformance.com

Cacao nibs (or powder): www.anthonysgood.com

Shelled hemp: www.canadahempfoods.com

Maca root powder: www.anthonysgood.com

Bee pollen: sunfood.com

Camu camu berry powder: sunfood.com

Ground cinnamon: Walmart

Vita Coco Organic Coconut Water: Walmart

Carrington Farms MCT Oil Powder: Walmart

Chlorella: www.microingredients.com

Cayenne Tincture: 1-800-HERB-DOC, though this ingredient is added as a liquid, not part of the dry mixture

When needed, I create a six-month for myself and keep in the freezer to preserve. Prudence suggests you try out these products first, as previously mentioned. Amazon and Walmart carry most of these products.

The cacao/cayenne combination in the drink mirrors an ancient Incan ceremonial elixir (41). *Be careful with the cayenne tincture at first!* At 250,000 HU (heat units), it deserves respect. Start off slowly…

Coconut water is the base liquid. I take my time consuming the morning drink, usually an hour or two. And I occasionally blend it into a smoothie, adding berries, bananas, Superfood Plus…

TYPICAL LUNCH

Lunch is *all fruit*: an avocado (only half if it's a big one), some raw almond butter with a few pieces of at least 78 percent dark chocolate, and a green banana and/or a green apple and/or half a grapefruit. The avocado will sustain.

TYPICAL DINNER

Is a salad consisting of greens, scallions, avocado, cultured veggies, and hot peppers. I top my salad with apple cider vinegar and olive oil or Mary's Oil Blend. I sprinkle minced garlic or ginger, sometimes both. After the salad, I'll have a bowl of soup, sometimes homemade, usually vegetarian (keeps longer in the fridge), sometimes canned. I like Amy's soups, organic, not over salted. I like sourdough toast with the soup and that terrific hard goat cheese from Trader Joe's, bereft of the A-1 casein protein in cow's milk that some find difficult to digest (21). During the evening, I will occasionally drink a cup of chamomile tea, as it naturally relaxes (28). A glass of red wine is also an option.

If I have a superpower, it's my ability to eat basically the same thing every day.

DESSERT?

Here's a great recipe for homemade ice cream, very simple and not too sweet. We'll call it *Piney Ponce's Ice Cream Special!* Put two cans of cream of coconut in a freezer-safe container, along with one tablespoon of vanilla, one tablespoon of maple syrup, and a pinch of sea salt. Shake it up, and put it in the freezer. After twenty minutes, check it and keep checking until it's ice cream! You can add fruit, cacao nibs, whatever you like, as long as it isn't sugar. You need vigilance, as leaving the mixture in too long will turn it to solid ice and you won't be able to consume it…

Occasionally on weekends, I will eat an aforementioned banana, almond butter, and avocado on sourdough for lunch, even gluten-free cereal for breakfast and lunch, sometimes eggs and sourdough toast. If I go out, it's usually Mexican food: pretty basic, low calorie, low glycemic, low gluten and my favorite, because of guacamole!

It is always my intention to eat healthy every day, every meal. I make it a point to tip the scale in favor of raw fruits, vegetables, superfoods and the other foods I suggest. I keep that commitment during holidays, though they are a challenge. If I consume something I'm not used to eating and feel a little off the next day, I'll take a Dr. Schulze's Intestinal Formula #1 to help remove the food from my system. Coconut water will pretty much do the same thing, as magnesium is a natural stool softener (50). If I'm invited to a gathering and feel I should bring food, I bring guacamole. It's a healthy choice and is a food everyone seems to like, as at evening's end there's usually none left. If dessert is necessary, I will bring Italian cheesecake, as it isn't as sweet as the regular type.

Aging is inevitable. We are all destined to grow old. Our bodies are programed to do so. We can try every health/longevity product, every new concept, but we will still grow old. There is grey, wiry hair growing on my arms; I'm freckling in strange places. I have a lizard neck I inherited from my father. The aesthetics of aging I will bear. But while I'm here, I want to live without so many physical complications. Stuff like aches and pains or old sports injuries will well up from time to time. But these aches and pains I vigorously address and I feel better.

I understand the sacrifice of giving up many of the foods we have enjoyed all our lives. But that food will no longer sustain us. The research supports this contention. And if you do change your diet, you'll probably catch grief, as I have, from friends and family for eating *weird food*. Perhaps the change in your degree of health will inspire them.

In so many of the books I've read, I thought it comical how the foods were described as *delicious* but actually tasted bad, at first. Now I crave those foods. You will get used to this food, even eventually prefer it.

> Eating raw, bitter foods…will actually change the taste of those foods…What you eat creates the signature in your salivary proteome, and those proteins modulate your sense of taste…If…people…try broccoli, (raw) greens… bitter foods, they'll taste better once they regulate these proteins (11).

Our intention must be to create a degree of health that needs no surgeries or procedures. To do this, the good food we consume must far outweigh the bad. We must wean ourselves from old, comfortable eating habits. Some may say modern medicine will save them even if they remain on the standard American diet. The medical system is designed to enable us to continue to eat the standard diet, but at what cost? So many of my family and friends have trusted and relied on this system with negative results.

I believe strongly in the habits I've written about in this book, so much so that I self-published it, and I'm not wealthy, nor am I particularly bold or outgoing. But this "is" crunch time. I'm going to get the word out. It works for me. Hopefully it will work for you too.

Good health is priceless. Tip the scale in favor of the foods and superfoods described in this book. Discard the foods and habits that do not support health.

It's simply a matter of choice.

ABOUT THE AUTHOR

Alan Larivee, BA, MA, is a writer, health enthusiast, and builder. He lives in southern Virginia.

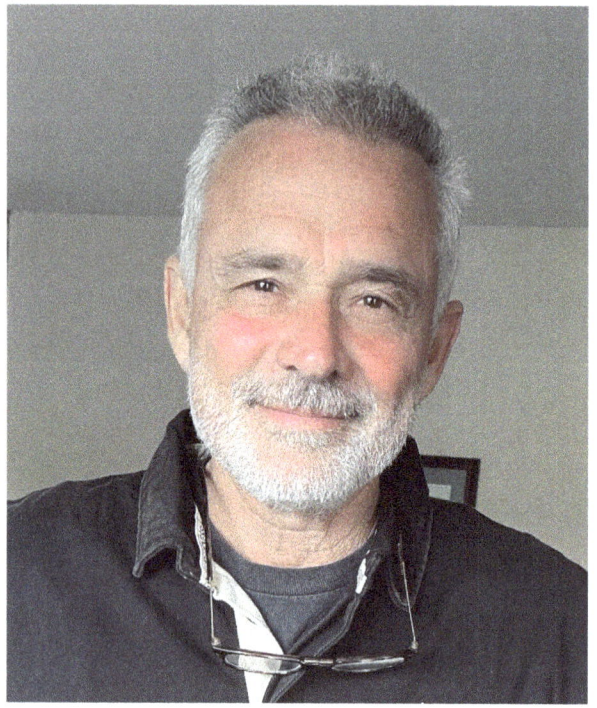

SUGGESTED READING

The Body Ecology Diet by Donna Gates

The Plant Paradox by Steven Gundry

Enter the Zone by Barry Sears

Superfoods, Eating for Beauty, Nature's First Law by David Wolfe

Earthing by Clint Ober, Martin Zucker, Steven Sinatra

The Promise of Sleep by William Dement

The Power of Now by Eckhart Tolle

Emotional Intelligence by Daniel Goleman

The Immortality Edge by Michael Fossel, Greta Blackburn, Dave Woynarowski

Breaking the Food Seduction by Neal Barnard

The Food Revolution by John Robbins

There Are No Incurable Diseases by Richard Schulze

Eat Fat to Lose Fat by Mary Enig and Sally Fallon

A Course in Miracles (No author cited)

There Is a Cure for Diabetes by Gabriel Cousins

ACKNOWLEDGMENTS

Special thanks to the folks from whom I've gathered so much knowledge, but also the ones who inspired:

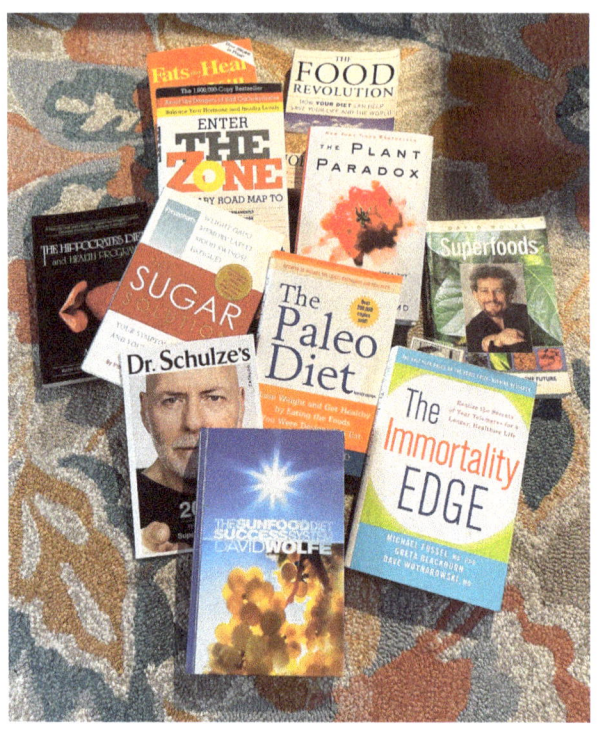

Barry Sears	Steven Gundry	Donna Gates
David Wolfe	Daniel Vitalis	Richard Schulze
Karen Panish	Mary Enig	Clint Ober
Andy Conklin	Ann Wigmore	Kent Eley
Neal Barnard	William Dement	John Robbins
Charlene Warren	Marci Wickesser	Chet Powers
Eckhart Tolle	Thomas Moore	Barkley Eley

And thanks to Weston Richards and all the folks at Palmetto
Publishing for the creation of this book!!!

WORKS CITED

1. Sears, Barry, PhD, and Bill Lawren, *Enter the Zone*, Harper Collins Publishing, 1995.

2. Wolfe, David, Steven Arlin, and Fouad Dini, *Nature's First Law: The Raw Food Diet*, Maul Publishing, 2003.

3. Erasmus, Udo, *Fats that Heal—Fats that Kill*, Alive Books, 1986.

4. Wolfe, David, *Superfoods: The Food and Medicine of the Future*, North Atlantic Books, 2009.

5. Staments, Paul, *Mycelium Running: How Mushrooms Can Help Save the World*, Ten Speed Press, 2005.

6. Gundry, Steven R., MD, *The Plant Paradox: The Hidden Dangers in "Healthy" Foods That Cause Disease and Weight Gain*, Harper Wave, 2017.

7. Ahmed, Serge H., Karine Guillem, and Youna Vandaele, Sugar Addiction: Pushing the Drug-Sugar Analogy to the Limit," National Library of Medicine, 2013.

8. Magalie, Lenoir, Fuschia Serre, Lauriane Cantin, Serge H. Ahmed, "Intense Sweetness Surpasses Cocaine Reward," Medline Plus, 2007.

9. Lippi, Giuseppe, "Meat Consumption and Cancer Risk: A Critical Review of Published Meta-Analysis," Elsevier, 2016.

10. Doyle, Derek, "Per Rectum: A History of Enemata," Royal College of Physicians of Edinburgh, 2005.

11. Martin, Laura, Kristen E. Kay, Ann-Marie Torregrossa, "Bitter-Induced Salivary Proteins Increase Detection of Quinine, but Not Sucrose," Chemical Senses, 2019.

12. Rabin, Roni Caryn, "Patients Must Be Warned of Breast Implant Risks, F.D.A. Says," *New York Times*, October, 2021.

13. Horstmeyer, Katie, RD, LDN, "Caffeine and the Elderly," Nutrition Care Systems, 2021.

14. Kubala, Jillian, MS, RD, "Eleven Reasons Why Sugar Is Bad for You," Healthline, 2018.

15. Schneider, Andrew, MD, "Tanglewood Foot Specialists," Houston, Texas.

16. Patel, Nammy, DDS, "The Dangers of Mercury Fillings: Why You Don't Want This in Your Mouth," Holistic Dentistry, 2018.

17. Howell, Edward, *Enzyme Nutrition: The Food Enzyme Concept*, Penguin Putnam, 1985.

18. Website, Surthrival.com, York, Maine.

19. *Break Bread With Us*. Blog.

20. Khait, Abi, "Stop Wearing Polyester Clothing," Beauty and Style Guide, 2019.

21. Zelman, Kathleen M., "Health Benefits of Goat Cheese," WebMD, September, 2024.

22. Whittel, Naomi, "6 Incredible Resveratrol Benefits For Your Health," naomi.com, 2022.

23. Gonzalez, S., T, Fernandez-Navarro, S. Arboleya, C.G. de los Reyes-Gavilan, N. Salazar, M. Gueimonde, "Fermented Dairy Foods: Impact on Intestinal Microbiota and Health Linked Biomarkers," Frontiers, 2019.

24. Ober, Clinton, Stephen T. Sinatra, and Martin Zucker, "Earthing: The Most Important Health Discovery Ever!," Basic Health Publications, 2014.

25. Epper, Margeaux, Pieying Yang, Richard W. Wagner, Lorenzo Coh, "Understanding the Link Between Sugar and Cancer: An Examination of the Preclinical and Clinical Evidence," National Library of Medicine, December, 2022.

26. No author cited, "What You Should Know About Candida and Drinking—Cheers to a Healthier Mardi Gras 2022!," AlignedModernHealth, March, 2022.

27. Fjeildberg, Grace, "Plant Power: Using Diet to Lower Cancer Risk," Mayo Clinic Health System, 2022.

28. Morales, Peter, and Marie Larraine, "What Are the Benefits of Chamomile Tea?," Medical News Today, 2023.

29. Rohmann, Emma, "Why Is Teflon So Bad and What Are the Alternatives?," EcoHOME, 2018.

30. Gates, Donna, and Linda Schatz, *The Body Ecology Diet,*, Hay House Publishers, 2011.

31. Bernstein, Elizabeth, "Foods that Help Battle Depression," *New York Times,* 2018.

32. Cheakalos, Christine, "Ten Reasons to Get a Dog When You're Over Fifty," AARP.

33. Rao, Harish, "Ghee Benefits: 10 Reasons Ghee Is a Superfood," Tin Star Foods, 2018.

34. Glicksman, Eve, "Your Brain on Guilt and Shame," BrainFacts, 2019.

35. Enig, Mary, and Sally Fallon, *Eat Fat to Lose Fat*, Penguin Publishing, 2006.

36. Price, Weston A, *Nutrition and Physical Degeneration*, Keats Publishing, 2003.

37. A Report from the Surgeon General, "Ten Health Effects of Smoking You Didn't Know About," American Lung Association, 2024.

38. Hahn, Joshua, Hafeez Ul Hassan Virk, Zhen Wang, Wei Hong W Tang, , "Cardiovascular Health Benefits of Theobromine in Cacao and Chocolate," AHAIASA Journals, November, 2021.

39. American Lung Association, "Toxic Air Pollutants," 2023.

40. Robinson, Haley, "The Health Benefits of Spicy Foods," Piedmont Healthcare, 2023.

41. Newman, Allen, "Preparing Ceremonial Cacao—A Guide for Lovers of Ancient Heart-Opening Chocolate," Ceremonial Cacao, 2018.

42. Coyne, Brian, "How Damaging Is Eating Late at Night?," Family Care Center Blog, 2018.

43. Shmerling, Robert, "Can Watching Sports Be Bad for Your Health?," Harvard Health Blog, 2019.

44. Saunders, Michael, "Study Finds Just 1 Drink Per Day Can Raise Blood Pressure Over Time," BU School of Public Health, August, 2023.

45. Jensen, Bernard, *Dr. Jensen's Guide to Body Chemistry and Nutrition*, Keats Publishing, 2000.

46. Satow, Roberta, "Depression and Dark Chocolate," *Psychology Today*, 2020.

47. Effective Integrative Healthcare, LLC, "13 Surprising Benefits of Getting a Chiropractic Adjustment," January 2022.

48. Reese, Mathieu, and Avi Varma, "How Can Viagra Effect Heart Health," Medical News Today, August, 2023.

49. Zhou, Cindy, "When and How Often Should You Brush Your Teeth," Mayo Clinic, July, 2023.

50. O'Neil, Terri, "Magnesium for Constipation," University of Michigan Medicine, March, 2021.

51. Martin, Laura, "How to Hold Your Liquor," WebMD, March, 2010.

52. Terry, Mary Beth, "Do Grilled Foods Cause Cancer," Columbia University Irving Medical Center, May, 2023.

53. Quote from the description overview in the TA-65 box that contained the TA-65 capsules.

54. Juber, Mahammad, "Health Benefits of Astaxanthin," WebMD, November, 2022.

55. Park, Jung Ha, Ji Hyun Moon, Hyena Ju Kim, Mi Her Kong, Sun Wan Oh, "Sedentary Lifestyle: Overview of Updated Evidence of Potential Health Risks," National Institute of Health, November, 2020.

56. Committees Conclusion, "The Health Effects of Cannabis and Cannabinoids," The National Academies of Sciences— Engineering—Medicine, January, 2021.

57. Raman, Ryan, and Marie Lorraine Johnson, "Top 11 Health Benefits of Bee Pollen," Healthiness, 2023.

58. Dement, William C., MD, PhD, and Christopher Vaughan, *The Promise of Sleep*, Random House, 1999.

59. Whits, Adrian, and Cathleen Marengo, "Can Aloe Vera Juice Treat IBS?," , Healthline, May, 2024.

60. More, William, and Zilpah Sheikh, "How Alcohol Affects Your Body,", WebMD, September, 2023.

61. Anding, Roberta, "Nutrition Made Clear," The Great Courses. 2009.

62. O'Brien, Sharon, "7 Evidence-Based Health of Camu Camu," Healthline, 2019.

63 Kandola, Aaron, and Natalie Olsen, "What Are the Benefits of Maca Root?," Medical News Today, December, 2023.

64. Schulze, Richard, *There Are No Incurable Diseases*, Natural Healing Publications, July, 1999.

65. Jennings, Kerri-Ann, "9 Impressive Health Benefits of Chlorella", Healthline, March, 2023.

66. Bell, Michael, "4 Surprising Health Benefits of Bee Pollen", Manukora, January, 2023.

67. Ware, Megan, "Potential Health Benefits of Spinach", Medical News Today, January, 2025.

68. Andrews, Alex, "Is Beer Gluten Free?" Small Beer, May, 2023.

69. Editorial Contributor, "Sunflower Oil: Is It Good For You?" WebMD, October, 2024.

70. Lopez-Alt, J. Kenji, "The Truth About Cast Iron Pans: 7 Myths That Need to Go Away", Serious Eats, November, 2024.

71. No author cited, "Things to Know Before Using Corningware Dishes in the Oven", Helton Tool and Home, September, 2023.

72. No author cited, "Make Floss Your Weapon Against Bacteria", Stensland Dental, July, 2013.

73. Clampolini, Mario, H. David Lovell-Smith, Timothy Kenealy, Riccardo Bianchi, "Hunger Can Be taught: Hunger Recognition Regulates Eating and Improves Energy Balance", International Journal of General Medicine, June, 2013.

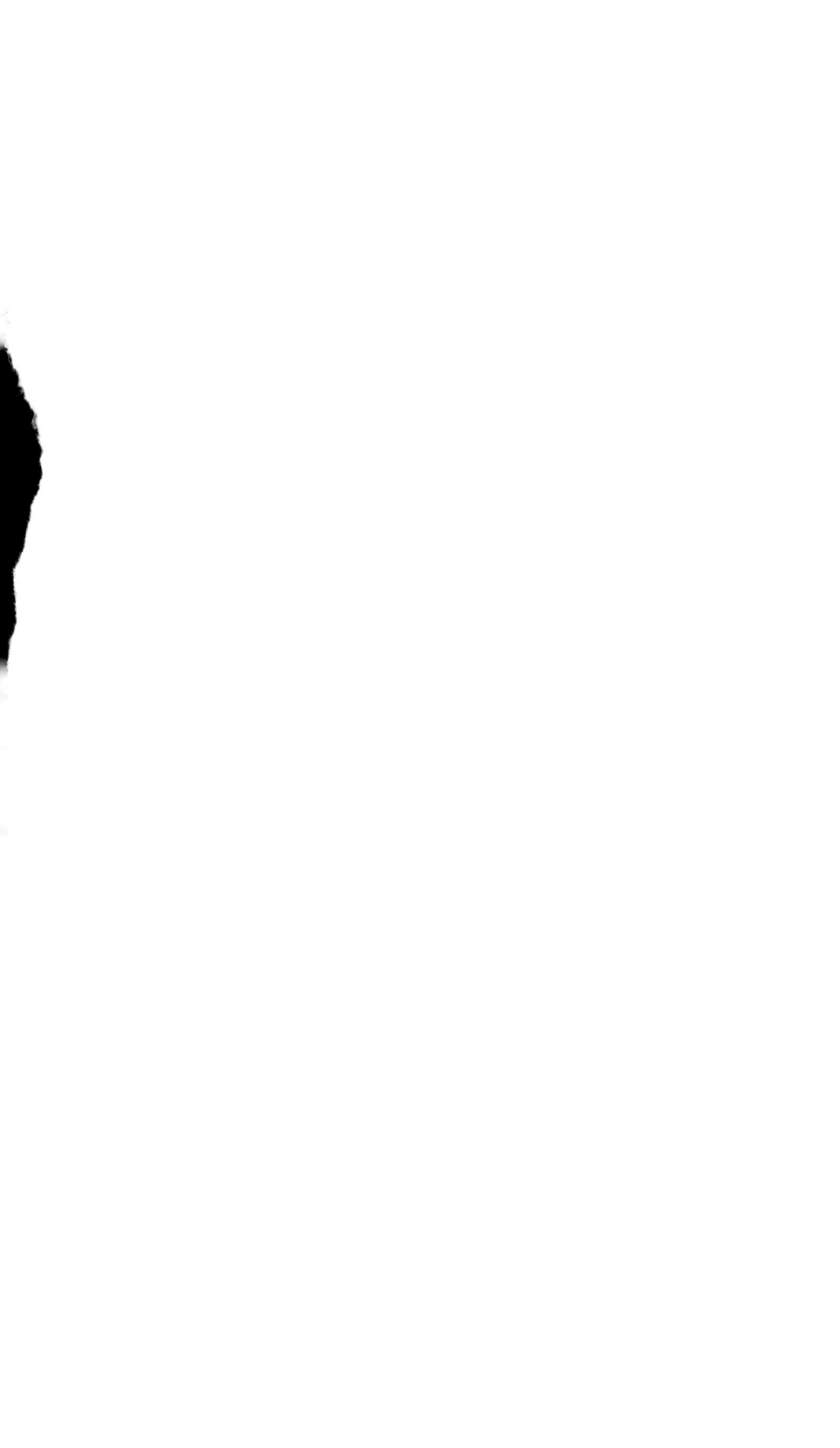

www.ingramcontent.com/pod-product-compliance
Lightning Source LLC
Chambersburg PA
CBHW041643240625
28656CB00046B/827